All the best with the rest of
your Midwifery training

Margy

XX

STANDING UP
FOR JAMES

D1331537

Published by Clarendon Publications Limited 2012
Suite 39, 9 Albert Embankment, London SE1 7HD

Copyright © Jane Raca 2012

Jane Raca has asserted her right under the Copyright, Designs and Patents Act 1988 to be identified as the author of this work.

All rights reserved. No part of this publication may be reproduced, stored in a retrieval system, or transmitted in any form or by any means electronic, mechanical, photocopying, recording or otherwise, without the prior permission of the copyright owner.

A CIP catalogue record for this book is available from the British Library.

PRINT   ISBN   978-0-9572887-0-6
EPUB   ISBN   978-0-9572887-2-0
MOBI   ISBN   978-0-9572887-1-3

Edited by **Susannah Straughan** - www.notreallyworking.co.uk

Printed and bound in the UK by **CPI Group (UK), Croydon, CR0 4YY**

Design and typesetting by **Devonshire-Jones Design**

Excerpt from The Thread taken from Landing Light © Don Paterson and reprinted by kind permission of Faber and Faber Ltd.

Excerpt from Walking Away by C. Day-Lewis taken from his Selected Poems, published by Enitharmon Press. Reproduced by kind permission of the Literary Estate of C. Day-Lewis.

Excerpts from records held by Birmingham City Council reproduced with their kind permission.

Excerpts from James's school records reproduced with the kind permission of Dame Hannah Rogers Trust and James's Birmingham school.

Excerpts from James's medical records reproduced by kind permission of Sandwell and West Birmingham Hospitals NHS Trust.

Contains public sector information licensed under the Open Government Licence v1.0.

Every effort has been made to trace copyright holders and to obtain their permission for the use of copyright material. The publisher apologises for any errors or omissions in the above list and would be grateful if notified of any corrections that should be incorporated in future reprints or editions of this book.

The publishers and the author believe that the legal references in this book are up to date at the time of publishing. However, any statements made as to the implications of any particular legislation or course of action are made purely for general guidance, and are not a substitute for independent professional advice. No liability can be accepted for loss incurred as a result of relying on statements in this book.

Papers used by CPI Group UK are from well-managed forests and other responsible sources.

Further copies of this book can be obtained via
www.standingupforjames.co.uk

Praise for Standing up for James

'I am sure this moving and well researched story mirrors the experience of many families with disabled children in Birmingham. The Council does not have the resources to fulfil all of its statutory obligations and so may avoid identifying a need which it cannot meet. Like other Councils across the country, it plays for time and space to protect its budgets. It relies on applicants' lack of knowledge about their rights, to achieve this. When it meets a strong applicant, it adopts the historic Russian military strategy of retreating, while it strengthens its position and weakens that of its opponent.

In Standing up for James, Jane Raca is raising issues of public policy and what sort of society we are becoming. These are questions that we cannot adequately answer, or are avoiding; in that sense she is standing up for all of us.'

Honorary Alderman Len Clark, former Birmingham City Councillor and chair of the Council's Inquiry into Protecting Children and Improving Children's Social Care, 2009.

'Social services departments have come under increased pressure to provide for children in need (including disabled children) at the same time that society demands that they respond urgently to children in need of protection. It is impossible for hard pressed social workers to do both well within limited or reducing resources. This book is a powerful description of the effect of that tension on one family and their struggle to get beyond it.'

Dr Anne Aukett, Consultant Paediatrician, Designated Doctor Safeguarding Children, Clinical Lead-Safeguarding Children, NHS West Midlands.

'A poignant account of the issues facing many families of children with special educational needs. This book will help parents by shining a light on some of the legal processes involved.'

Clive Rawlings, specialist education law barrister, Hardwicke Chambers.

For my mother and my husband,
without whom I wouldn't still be here.

For the staff at Birmingham City Hospital,
without whom James wouldn't still be here.

For the staff at Dame Hannah Rogers Trust
who set him free.

STANDING UP
FOR JAMES

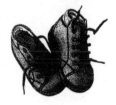

Jane Raca

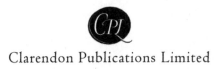

Clarendon Publications Limited

CONTENTS

Foreword
ROSA MONCKTON
STANDING UP FOR JAMES

Jane Raca has written a very important book, which should be required reading for every MP, for every person in a local authority who has anything to do with providing services for disabled children, and for any doctor or nurse charged with their care. Parents of disabled children will be all too familiar with the terrible journey that can unfold. However, everyone should read this book, to understand how you can go from thinking you are in control of your life, to wanting to end it.

Jane chronicles with devastating frankness the story of her son's premature birth at 25 weeks, to his arrival at Dame Hannah Rogers School for a residential placement at the age of eight.

James has cerebral palsy and autism. He is epileptic, doubly incontinent, cannot walk or talk, and has severe learning disabilities. Jane's family should have received immediate and unquestioning support from the appropriate services. This book takes us each step of the way with Jane in her fight to get what her child needed, and what was his by legal right.

She reveals the labyrinthine complexities of a system which, we must believe, was designed to help a disabled child, but which is paralysed by bureaucracy, and lacking any form of common sense.

Jane writes in a clear-headed way about the effect that having a disabled child had on her health, her other children and her relationship with her husband. A child like James requires 24-hour care, which implicitly means that there can be no time for anyone else, least of all for Jane. She describes with searing honesty her descent into chronic depression, and the fight that she had to save her marriage.

One reads with utter disbelief that Jane and her husband Andrew had to go to an advocate to try and get respite care from social services. The advocate assured them that they would qualify as top priority for respite. However, three months after they were told they were eligible for the funding, they were told that they would have to wait for two years until James was seven, before they got any respite from anywhere.

They appealed, and it took three months to get a response. The social worker rang to arrange a date, but she didn't turn up. It took them ten months to get 24 days' respite a year. The description of the first weekend break with their two other children makes almost unbearable reading: 'The other children were coming alive with something they had never known. It was at once too much and too little.'

The extraordinary love that Jane has for her son is manifest when she decides that the best thing for him, for her and the whole family would be for him to be in residential care. She sent the local authority a ten-page essay entitled 'Life with James', describing what it was like to look after him 24 hours a day. There was no response. 'Nothing happened' is a phrase that is repeated in this chapter. They end up in court. Andrew, Jane's husband, stands up and says: 'James likes me to walk him to the window, and he puts his hand on it and looks at me. And I say "Yes James, it's cold." Then he puts his hand on the radiator and looks at me again. And I say "Yes James, it's hot." He knows the difference between hot and cold. And he wants to hear me say it because he can't say it. He's very bright, but we can't give him what he needs at home. So we are showing our love for him by coming to this tribunal and asking for him to go to Dame Hannah Rogers School.'

Finally they won their case, and James is now being

professionally looked after. But as Jane says: 'There should be a clear, open pathway for children like James. What higher priority for state spending could there be?'

However this is not a depressing book. On the contrary, Jane's strength, intelligence and fighting spirit win through, and she uses her training as a lawyer to fight back against the system which treats people like her son so cruelly.

There is a description of Jane taking James into a shop to buy a birthday card for her mother. James was wailing, flailing his arms, hitting his head and biting his hand. Onlookers stared in disbelief, but one woman went up to the counter, made a purchase and turned round to Jane, saying: 'This is for you, you are doing a wonderful job.' It was a tiny teddy wearing a T-shirt which said: 'World's no. 1 Mum!' Read this book. She is.

Rosa Monckton

Rosa Monckton is President of KIDS (a national charity which cares for children with disabilities and their families), and Patron of several other children's charities. These include Downside Up (a Moscow-based charity for children with Down's syndrome), and Acorns Children's Hospice. She is actively involved in the Bulgarian Abandoned Children's Trust. She writes for *The Daily Mail* newspaper, and has presented three BBC TV documentaries on children and young adults with disabilities in Britain. She is married to journalist Dominic Lawson, and has two daughters, one of whom has Down's syndrome.

Introduction
TWO WORLDS

Until I was 36, I lived in what I thought was the normal world. I was a solicitor with a happy marriage, a healthy toddler and a nice house. Then in 1999 my second child James was born at 25 weeks, with extensive brain damage, and I entered the disabled world.

It began with a four-month fight in hospital for James's life. When he survived, we pressed his consultants to tell us what he would be like – what he would be able to do or not do. They could only guess.

When he came home, we faced a slowly emerging picture of a boy who couldn't walk, talk or use his left hand. He was also handsome, clever and funny. Everyone who cared for him fell in love with him, and he fell in love back.

As he grew older, he began to show signs of unusual behaviour. He hated to leave the house except to go to school. He was only happy when watching clips of *Teletubbies* over and over again. He would eat nothing but ham sandwiches and crisps. We overlooked these foibles, uneasy about what they might mean. All small children had tantrums and food fads, didn't they? But the behaviour crossed the line between the normal and disabled worlds and heralded another devastating diagnosis: James was severely autistic.

Before long he began to attack us on a regular basis. He separated his food into piles of different things before eating it. He also ate his own faeces. He woke at 4am almost every day and shouted for hours. We became stupefied zombies.

When James was five, we sat in front of his consultant and wept at the unbearable lives we now led. She referred us to the social care department of Birmingham City Council, and so began the final transformation of two confident professionals into two broken people who were tremblingly dependent on the state to save them.

What followed is the reason I have written this book. I was so shocked by the inadequacies of the system that greeted us that I felt compelled to do something about it. I have taken a deep breath, put my privacy to one side and given a personal account of my family's experience, to try and raise awareness of what is going on.

In her foreword, Rosa Monckton has referred to what happened to us. But we are not alone. All over the UK, parents of disabled children are feeling tortured in their homes by lack of sleep and respite, and by the sheer unremitting responsibility they bear.

Their children aren't getting the physiotherapy they require, so their limbs are seizing up, leading to a lifetime of immobility and pain. Siblings are losing their childhoods because they're being deprived of parental attention and basic life opportunities, or turned into little carers. Some women have even been driven to kill themselves and their children out of sheer despair and exhaustion.

Throughout the book I have referred to normal or ordinary people, as opposed to disabled people. This isn't very politically correct, because the philosophy in the disabled world is that there is no such thing as normal – there are just people, with their different needs and abilities. I agree with that philosophy. I see it as an extension of the view that it doesn't matter what language you speak, how you dress, or what colour your skin is – you are a human being.

However, in talking about children who are as extremely disabled as James, I had to find some context that everyone could easily understand. That is what mattered, not the semantics of disability.

Although I have changed some names at the request of the people described, everything in this story really happened.

Chapter 1
LIFE BEFORE JAMES

It was the height of the Thatcher years, and for me it really felt as if the streets ran with champagne. I had a flat in Dulwich, a boyfriend who was a parliamentary candidate and a salary which kept going up every six months. I thought I was very clever and important. Almost everyone I knew then was young and successful like me, and I wasn't very interested in those who weren't. I didn't notice people in wheelchairs. If I saw someone in the street with an obvious mental disability I would feel embarrassed, lower my eyes and move away.

I didn't have a privileged childhood. My parents separated when I was 12 and my father, a software consultant, moved to Los Angeles. My mother worked as a secretary to support my sister and me. I was bright, though, and ended up at Bristol University reading Law. By the late 1980s I was a solicitor in a central London practice.

In the day, I would take the tube to work, wearing brightly coloured suits with large shoulder pads and gold buttons. As my career progressed, I was involved with newsworthy cases.

There was Lord Brocket, who buried his collection of classic cars in the grounds of his stately home, to claim the insurance money. Even more notorious was Robert Maxwell, who mysteriously fell off his yacht, *The Lady Ghislaine*, and drowned. It later emerged that he had raided the pension fund of Mirror Group Newspapers to keep his businesses afloat.

In the evenings, I would often meet with colleagues in Covent Garden or go to functions with my boyfriend, Andrew. We listened to Kenneth Clarke and Chris Patten at our annual dinners in Southwark. There was a cocktail party at the Foreign Office, where glamorous women whisked us from one introduction to another, until we were giddy. We went to a reception with Norman Lamont, then Chancellor of the Exchequer, where I drank two glasses of Sancerre on an empty stomach and started to advise him on restructuring the mortgage system.

When Andrew and I got engaged, we decided to move out of London. We had a family life in mind and somehow that didn't go with underground stations and rush hour on Waterloo Bridge.

I joined a national law firm based in the Midlands and started on the long road to a partnership. I tried to plot a long path to motherhood beside it. I drew little charts showing how late I could wait to get promoted before I had baby number one. I even calculated the best month of the year to get pregnant, so that it didn't clash with the assessment process. I really thought I was in control of my life.

By 1996 I was a partner in the litigation department. At parties when I was asked what I did for a living I used to say, 'I sue people'. Then a year later my first child, Tom, was born.

I had no experience of babies or children – there had been none in my family for years. I was knocked sideways by the intensity of parental love and the sense of responsibility for this tiny person. I was also horrified by the chaotic turn that domestic life had taken. How could such a little scrap generate piles of washing the size of African anthills, or have the audacity to wake me several times a night for a breast-feed? After a few days Andrew did late evening duty, so that if I went to bed at 8pm I could at least get four hours of unbroken sleep. During these times he fed Tom a bottle and derived a great deal of fatherly satisfaction from making him burp.

I did the lion's share of looking after Tom, as I was on

maternity leave and Andrew had a long commute to work. He was also, rather inconveniently, campaigning in a general election. I tried accompanying him on the campaign trail, taking Tom in a Moses basket. These long, late trips were just too tiring, though, so I reverted to staying at home. I felt rather isolated as my mother was nursing my ill and elderly grandmother; my sister worked full time and knew even less about babies than I did. Both lived miles away. Andrew's mother, who was Polish and lived nearer, supported me with home-made chicken soup and an encyclopaedic knowledge of treatments for infant ailments.

When Tom was four months old, with considerable relief I handed him over to a nanny and went back to work full time. The nanny was, I reasoned, far more qualified than I to look after him. After all, she had a certificate and years of experience, whereas I was just a beginner. I enjoyed putting my suit on and escaping from the isolation and mess of the house, back to my familiar office full of orderly files. Brought up on a diet of *Cosmopolitan* magazine and Germaine Greer, it hadn't crossed my mind to sideline my career to look after my baby. I had always intended to have both. The realisation that while this might be possible it wasn't necessarily desirable, took a while to sink in.

The first milestone I missed was Tom speaking. The nanny rang me when I was in a meeting to tell me that he had said 'Yum', when being fed a banana. At the time I thought 'Oh good, I'll hear it when I get home.' If I'd known then how long I would wait in vain for James to utter any word at all, I would not have taken Tom's first one for granted.

For Tom's first birthday the nanny organised a party at an indoor play area, with a gang of other nannies and their charges. I sneaked away from work to be there for an hour, feeling very much the outsider because everyone else knew each other. A deep unease came over me as I remembered my childhood parties at home, with jelly in paper bowls, games like pass the parcel and, most of all, mothers. When Tom cried it was the nanny, not me, who rocked him to sleep.

Then there were his vaccinations. I had taken Tom for his first set while I was on maternity leave. I had held him as the needle made a sharp and unexpected scratch, and soothed him afterwards while he cried with pain and shock. Now he'd reached 12 months, I realised that the nanny would have to take him for the second set. I felt an inward dismay; surely this comforting was not something I should be subcontracting? After James was born I was there for all of his medical procedures, at least until he went to Dame Hannah Rogers School. In the early years, those appointments were James's milestones, instead of walking and talking.

The uneasy feeling about being absent from much of Tom's life was resolved when we decided we had to move nearer to Andrew's job. His lengthy commute on top of Tom's 5am starts had become intolerable for him. I didn't want to commute either, so the move would mean I had to look for another job. Suddenly I realised how very much I didn't want to do that. I wanted to spend more time with Tom and I wanted another baby! We agreed that I would give up work for a while and we would try.

By the time we moved into our new house in Birmingham, I was raring to start my life as a full-time mum. However, when I watched Andrew drive the nanny to the station for the last time and glimpsed her face through the back of the retreating car, I was overcome by panic. I had to turn and face the empty house with Tom, now 18 months old, my sole responsibility.

The first days were awful. I knew no one and I began to realise the full extent to which I didn't know Tom. I had fondly hoped I might read the newspaper each morning while he played with his train set. Instead, I quickly found that I had to join in and build new and exciting track configurations, or else my attempts to read were cruelly sabotaged. I realised that I needed a 'mummy network'.

I had noticed a sign outside the local church advertising a toddler group. 'Pram Pushers' sounded like a name left over from the 1950s, which no one had thought to change. But it was a relief to share cups of weak instant coffee with other mums, although I found some of the uninhibited discussions about children's toilet habits embarrassing. We compared notes on the various stages of development which our offspring had reached, though these sometimes became a little competitive.

Tom was bright, able to talk quite well and to operate the most complex toys. How proud I was of this, never imagining that when I took James to the same group in later years, he wouldn't even be able to throw a ball.

After a few weeks there were about ten mums I could arrange to see for a coffee and a chat, while our toddlers built brick towers around our feet. During our picnics and excursions to adventure playgrounds and animal farms, I occasionally thought back to the office. While I missed my salary, I had no wish to return.

Andrew and I had been trying for another baby since we moved house and nothing had happened. I started to have scans of my monthly cycle to make sure there were no problems. On the second scan the nurse's face broke into a broad grin. She showed me a little white blob on the monitor. 'Congratulations' she said. 'You won't need to see me any more, you're pregnant!'

We had not had any antenatal testing done with Tom, unable to bear the idea that we might lose him, as the only tests available then carried a risk of miscarriage. Now we could have a non-invasive test to find out if there was a greater than normal chance of the baby having Down's syndrome. This was the most common disability for a child, given my age. We agreed that we wanted to be prepared, but that whatever the result we would have the baby. When we learned that the risk was very low, we sighed with relief and moved on from this brief glimpse into the dark world of disability.

Underneath it all, we were sure that it would never happen to us.

Chapter 2
TSUNAMI

'Jamie made his landing in the world
so hard he ploughed straight back into the earth.
They caught him by the thread of his one breath
and pulled him up. They don't know how it held.' [1]

I never was good at being pregnant, but looking back on
it something was going terribly wrong in the fifth month of
carrying James.

I had an episode of cramping pain, although this passed
and the hospital confirmed that all was well. So we went
ahead with our planned holiday to Yorkshire.

We had taken a reluctant decision to stay in England
rather than to go somewhere more exotic. Afternoon teas in
grey stone towns didn't give us a holiday high – we wanted
to be sipping rosé wine in French street cafés. However, we
had been to Poland when I was pregnant with Tom and I
had felt vulnerable, being so far from home.

As Tom was still an early riser, our days started horribly
early. By 9am we'd already be making sandcastles at Whitby
Bay. We chuffed around on steam railways, wandered round
parks and sat in cafés eating those filling Yorkshire teas. In
all outward respects it was exactly the right sort of holiday
to take with a toddler and a baby on the way.

But I was feeling more and more lethargic. My hair had
the consistency of straw. I had become pale and tired, only
able to walk a few steps before needing to sit down. Photos
from that time show that James was lying ominously low. If
the birth had been due sooner I would have been worried.
But I was only 24 weeks pregnant. To me he was just a half

[1] *Excerpt from The Thread, taken from Landing Light © Don Paterson,*
reprinted by kind permission of Faber and Faber Ltd.

baked biscuit, cooking nicely. If I was feeling tired and had a few pains, then surely that was normal?

The photos from that holiday are poignant. In them my eyes shine with the comfortable innocence of someone for whom life has always been both predictable and fair. I could not have imagined the tsunami which was about to roar through my emotional landscape, leaving it strewn with wreckage and unrecognisable.

As if to nod to our wisdom in not going abroad, fate held back from delivering James until the day after we came home from Yorkshire. (We later realised that if we had gone to France, I would have been on the overnight sleeper train somewhere around Lyon.) My waters broke, and in a state of shock I calmly told Andrew that he would have to look after Tom while I drove myself to hospital. Equally in shock, Andrew protested that he had to go to work.

I got to the hospital only to find that there were no free parking spaces except for 20-minute stay only bays. I remember wondering how long I would need to be there and being unable to continue with that thought. I left the car in short stay anyway and went into the maternity unit, where I was immediately admitted.

The door was flung open and an important-looking consultant strode in followed by a team of at least four staff. Unfortunately I don't remember anything that was said, except that I would need to be moved to another hospital. The hospital I was in was world renowned, world class and modern. The one the consultant wanted to send me to was Victorian, smelly and in a dodgy part of town.

I didn't want to go anywhere, but when I protested, in that strident way so common in middle-class English women, a rather scathing sister told me that if I preferred, there was a bed available for me in Edinburgh. (I didn't know then that sometimes pregnant mothers are transferred all over the UK to give birth, wherever there is a neonatal cot available for their baby.) By this time the shock had deepened and my mind had begun to spin clouds of cotton wool around itself. I could not understand that I was going to give birth and that the hospital needed a cot in intensive care for my son. In my mind he was not due for another 15 weeks, so whatever was going to happen, birth was not it.

I was then put on a stretcher in an ambulance to travel to the Victorian hospital. I later read in James's medical notes that this was quaintly called an 'intra-uterine transfer'.

The paramedic and the nurse who travelled with me chatted about football, the weather and hospital food. Every now and then they would ask if I was all right. I nodded silently. My whole body felt like a sob. If I allowed myself to speak I would cry. If I cried, the terror which was building inside me would be let out and I would not know what to do with it.

*

The cotton wool continued to weave itself in my head, so by the time I arrived at Birmingham's City Hospital I was almost insensible. They gave me my own room. It was large and painted in a sickly powder pink. A clock on the wall ticked loudly, as the second hand moved around. The hand quivered slightly, as if it were being liberated with each passing second. There was a water stain on the ceiling, and I stared at it and listened to the clock without thinking of anything.

Eventually a consultant came in. This was Miss D, who sailed, rather than strode. It was she who explained to me, finally, the details of what was happening: labour was inevitable, they couldn't stop it and I would give birth to my son soon. In the meantime I was on complete bed rest and it was my job to stay pregnant for as long as possible. Every day counted.

This was the first time anyone had talked to me about the baby in a meaningful way. The cotton wool parted for a moment. I was hearing something which justified throwing off the mental duvet. 'Do you mean he's not going to die?' I asked. Miss D looked at me, 'Babies born at 24 weeks have a 50 per cent chance of survival.'

I finally comprehended the situation I was in. I was going to give birth, but not necessarily now, and the baby wouldn't necessarily die. In fact, he might very well live.

From that moment on, everything changed. I had assumed under the cotton wool of shock that I had lost the baby. Now I had real hope. All of the tension turned into immutable resolve. I was not going to move from my bed and he was going to live.

Miss D asked me if we had a name for him and I told her yes, it was going to be James. It was fortunate that Andrew and I had agreed the name a few days earlier, as we wouldn't have been capable of doing so now. For the four months that James was there, the hospital whiteboard in the neonatal unit had several new admissions labelled 'Jane Doe' or 'John Doe', where stupefied parents had still to decide what to call their children.

Andrew eventually arrived. He had taken Tom to stay with Polish Grandma, 'Babcia'. This was not a happy arrangement, as she had never looked after him on her own before, particularly overnight. Tom didn't know her very well, and he had never been apart from me. However, we needed help immediately and she was nearest. We were in such shock we didn't think to ask my family to come from further away, although I'm sure they would have done.

After about 24 hours, James decided he had had enough of lying inside this still and anxious mummy, and contractions began. I would have lain in that ward for weeks to keep him safe, but it was completely outside my control and the hospital system geared up for birth.

I was taken into the delivery suite. We noticed that in the corner of the room was a machine. It looked like my mother's old Belling cooker and had the rather chilling name of Resuscitaire. On close inspection, Andrew noticed a label that said 'Not to be used on infants under 1.5kg'. We were sufficiently focused to point out this potential problem to the nurses, who removed it and brought in a smaller version.

I was given an epidural, as it would slow the birth down and allow the doctors more control. But this worked too well, so I was then given Syntocinon to speed things up. Meanwhile Andrew had become overwhelmed and desperately hungry. The hospital canteen had closed as it was about 10pm, so I sent him off to get a takeaway pizza. While he was gone, I felt a strange sensation and the midwife told me that she could see James's feet – he was in breach position.

I was very scared of what James would be like, being born so early. Images of foetuses from anti-abortion campaigns dangled in front of my eyes, and I couldn't bring myself to picture, never mind touch, the person who was being born. I later found out that James's feet had become very cold as the birth was so slow, and it had taken hours to warm them up. How I wish I had held those tiny feet, to reassure my son that I was there for him from the start!

Andrew returned from his pizza and suddenly the room was full of people. With the combined effects of the epidural and his tiny size, I don't remember the exact moment of James's birth. I just became aware that everyone had stopped concentrating on me.

There was no sound from James, who was eventually wheeled in an incubator to the neonatal unit, accompanied by an entourage of staff, leaving me behind. I later learnt from Andrew that he hadn't known whether to be with me or James, but he had eventually gone with his son, the main lead in this drama.

My part in the crisis over, my husband and baby gone, I began to lie back and take stock. But I had forgotten about the placenta. Designed to remain part of me for the next

15 weeks, it wouldn't come out. Two midwives tugged and teased at it, but it felt as though they were taking out my entrails. I had been brave for a long time, but I was now very tired and all my resources were spent. I lost control of myself completely, and a harpy inside me, who I had never met before, took over. I screamed at the nurses to 'Just get the bloody thing out!', and that I wanted to die. The epidural had worn off and I was in agony. Then Andrew reappeared, took one look at me and went to find the doctor.

The epidural was topped up and I was taken into theatre. There was more tugging. A surgeon was trying to tell me what he was doing. I found his African accent so broad that I couldn't understand anything he was saying. I fell asleep and was woken immediately by the anaesthetist, concerned that I had passed out. Eventually it was over, and I was wheeled out to recovery.

I had not eaten or slept for two days. I began to retch with hunger, exhaustion and shock. I didn't think it was possible to be alive and to feel any lower.

After a brief sleep and a piece of cold hospital toast with margarine, I went to see James. I was taken in a wheelchair because of the epidural; it wasn't safe to walk as I couldn't completely feel my legs yet.

It was helpful not to have to make any physical effort, but just to be pushed. Since I had driven myself to the first hospital three days earlier, I hadn't walked anywhere. I had completely lost control of my life, so it felt fitting. I don't think I would have been able to take myself from my bed in the maternity ward to the wing which housed the neonatal unit: I was too scared of what I might find there.

I was wheeled into lifts and along what seemed to be acres of green, echoing corridors. I remember the smell which filled them, of disinfectant mixed with the day's hot catering. Eventually we arrived at a heavy, security-coded door, with a small glass panel.

There was a nurse looking through it, waiting to let me

in, and she took me straight ahead to the intensive care ward where James was, ventilated and in an incubator. As I was wheeled in, I took one look and had to beg to be taken out. I had caught a glimpse of a tiny red frog in a plastic box, obscured by a forest of tubes.

Later in the day, I was summoned to see the consultant on duty. Dr B didn't sail or stride, he melted into a room.

I wasn't expecting what he said next. James had had a haemorrhage in the fluid-filled cavities called ventricles on both sides of his brain. If the bleeding continued, it would burst the walls of the ventricles and spill onto the brain tissue. This would deprive his brain of oxygen and cause brain damage, possibly death. There was nothing they could do, we would just have to sit and wait. The first 72 hours were critical. If James got through that, his chances of survival would increase.

Dr B asked me if I had understood what he had said, and I said I had. I just managed to leave the room and get back to my bed before I broke down. When Andrew arrived, I was unable to tell him the news, so Dr B had to repeat it to both of us.

We decided to write to everyone we knew, to tell them that James had been born. Andrew needed something to fend off all the concerned phone calls, which were already beginning and were so awful to deal with.

Although the note was only a few lines long, we were in such shock that it took us two hours to compose. We told people that James had been born prematurely, but not about the brain damage. That wasn't a conscious decision, but we were simply unable to comprehend what Dr B had said. Also, at that time all we cared about was that James lived. Nothing else mattered.

The nurses asked us if we were religious and did we want James baptised? They thought it might be a 'good idea'. Since he only had a 50 per cent chance of surviving, we saw what they meant. That night, because the Anglican vicar from our church was in the south of France, and no one else was available, a priest came from a local Catholic church instead.

He stood over James's incubator, saying the ancient words we had heard before at christenings, about being welcomed into the light – words which had never seemed so powerful. His surplice was stained with gravy and he was grumpy and monotone, but we wept with relief when he had finished the ceremony. Andrew went home alone to look after Tom, as I couldn't bear to leave the hospital.

In those first few days, when James's life was really at risk, I experienced the absolute terror of a parent facing the loss of a child. Black fear swamped me. James would be beyond my ability to comfort him. I had always been a 'Christmas Christian', now I reached out to the only Being I could think of who could possibly watch over James in the swirling darkness of death. I prayed to God fervently, passionately and with total humility.

The ventricles in James's brain did burst, destroying most of the right side of his brain and part of his left. But after 72 hours he was still alive and stable, and I began to experience the most intense joy I had ever known.

*

As I became more and more able to look at James, I saw that he was like a skinned rabbit, red and shiny and not human. His birth weight had been 800 grams, although 1lb 12oz had more meaning for me, as I could compare it to blocks of butter.

The nurses began gently to teach me about his condition and how to do his 'cares'. This meant changing and cleaning him and his sheets, as with any baby. But with James it all had to be done with military precision and surgical cleanliness. My hands were disinfected and then I would insert a tiny cotton bud through the portholes of the incubator, taking care not to let it touch anything but James. He had doll-size nappies which I could change, but there were too many tubes going into his body to make it possible to dress him.

After a couple of days in hospital to recover from the birth I was told I could go home. At first I couldn't contemplate leaving. I felt that the incubator was in effect my womb, and that James was still part of me, yet to be born. That feeling was reinforced by the medical staff, who treated the babies based on their projected due dates. Each week that went by James would get nearer to his due date, and if he survived, he would come home around the time he should have been born.

Eventually though, I realised that I had to escape from the intensity of the hospital, its smells and noise and also to see Tom, who had been without me for nearly a week. The nurses promised to ring me at any time 24 hours a day if there was any change, and I resolved to keep my phone next to my pillow at night.

Returning home was at once a source of devastation and relief. I had come back without my baby, but I had returned to my toddler. Thanks to the note Andrew had sent out, people knew what had happened. Their response was immediate. Everyone wrote back to us. We even had letters from people we barely knew, who had heard the news second hand.

The barriers and social niceties just went. People seemed to have sat down, wherever they were, and written on whatever was at hand. There was paper torn from a notebook, even a piece of graph paper. They wrote urgently and with the most compassionate words their particular style could find. They were what we needed. Our legs had been cut from under us and we had no strength.

One friend had a Mass dedicated to James. We later found out that other people had arranged for prayers to be said in their local churches. Sometimes we would open the front door to find a dish of freshly cooked pasta or some cakes, which a kind neighbour had left without disturbing us. Thank goodness I had made some friends before this happened. Many of them were vegetarians, and though Andrew was a voracious carnivore, he gratefully devoured anonymously donated dishes of Quorn chilli and cauliflower cheese.

The umbilical cord may have been cut at birth, but to me it stretched from home to the neonatal unit two miles away. How lucky I was not to be in a hospital in Edinburgh! I put poor bewildered Tom into nursery and began a daily routine of visiting the hospital.

After a little while James was able to stop receiving nutrition via a drip and to tolerate breast milk, which I had been expressing since birth for the nurses to freeze. He still couldn't suck, so he had to receive it through a tube which went down his nostril into his stomach. The nurses couldn't stop praising me for breast-feeding, and they made me feel like a clever schoolgirl. I had never been so aware before of the benefits of breast milk, the antibodies and sterility. I was pleased to be able to do something for James, as I couldn't cuddle him or bathe him. I so missed the sense of connecting with him, of him sucking my breast and pulling the milk out of me. I used to cry with the loss of that feeling.

There was a curtain screen around the breast pump in the neonatal unit, which is etched on my memory. It was made of thick white cotton with brightly coloured clowns in red, green, yellow and blue. They were doing somersaults and juggling, and their jollity was an insult to the feelings I was going through. I used to stare at them while the breast pump went thump, suck, thump, suck. I saw the same curtain in another hospital several years later: it must have been an NHS bulk buy. Even though I had long ceased breast-feeding, I swear I could feel the letdown when I saw those curtains!

One nurse endeared herself to us from the start. Karen was a small Malaysian woman with short black hair, who introduced herself as James's lead nurse. She looked at me and Andrew sternly, and explained that James had better behave because she was 'very bossy'. She made us feel as if we had better behave too. There would be no mistakes when Karen was on the ward.

All the nurses had a way of humanising the babies, which took away some of the distress caused to their parents by the strange environment in which they existed. There were no cries to be heard; only the quiet talk of the staff and the beeping of the machines which dominated the room. One nurse told me how handsome she thought James was, and greeted him with 'Hello sexy'. Another would go up to his incubator and report our early morning telephone calls to him, when we rang to see how he was.

I still found my emotions fluctuating violently between ecstasy that he was alive, and shock at what had happened. I remember saying arrogantly to the registrar, 'Things like this don't happen to people like me.' She replied earnestly that premature babies happened across all age groups and social classes and there was often no identified cause.

At first James slept on synthetic sheepskin fleeces, and looked rather biblical, swathed inside his incubator. As he grew bigger, by a few grams each day, the sheepskin was taken for more needy babies and replaced with sheets. I noticed that sometimes these were brushed cotton – very soft and comforting – but at other times they were thin, flat and cold looking. I was hypersensitive to every aspect of James's environment – something which has never left me. This was partly because he was so vulnerable, but also because I could do so little for him myself. I bought my own brushed cotton sheets and took them home to wash, rather than leave them to the hospital laundry. Once James could wear clothes, I also began to buy premature baby clothes, instead of using the hospital ones. Many of the hospital clothes were knitted or crocheted by kindly old ladies, and got caught in James's fingers.

Karen taught me to read the monitors that showed James's heart rate and oxygen levels. The whole of his stay in hospital was really a war with oxygen. He would progress through three parts of the neonatal unit, depending on how stable he was. In intensive care, the babies were on ventilators. When they graduated to the high dependency ward they would slowly be introduced to oxygen fed via small nasal prongs. Eventually, when they could start to be weaned off oxygen altogether, they would be moved to the cot nursery, for fattening up prior to coming home.

While the babies were dependent on oxygen, they would be hooked up to monitors, which would beep when the oxygen level in their blood dipped. Sometimes James would become bradycardic, when his heart beat very slowly, triggering the monitors. The nurses called this 'having a braddy'. I would leap up in fear, looking for someone to help. But they taught me to 'look at the baby, not the monitor'. Gradually, I noticed that James usually recovered from the braddy by himself, although sometimes they needed to turn the oxygen supply up.

Once, the lesson to 'look at the baby' really paid off when I noticed James's lips turning blue, even though no alarm went off at first. The nurses must have seen my face and came rushing over. The ventilator tube in James's throat had slipped, so he was hardly getting any oxygen, even though the ventilator machine was puffing away. The head of the unit came over and I sensed the rising panic among the staff. She began reciting her training out loud as she corrected the position of the tube. Gradually James's face turned back from deep blue to dusky pink.

Apart from doing his 'cares' I was allowed to touch James briefly, by stroking his temples extremely gently. I found it very moving when the monitors showed that his heart rate slowed in response, as he relaxed.

Andrew used to come and hug the incubator, as if it were James. He made a tape of the family's voices for James, to remind him of what he would be hearing if he were at home.

When James was six days old, I came in to find the nurses and a young, unsmiling doctor waiting for me. She had long black hair and hard eyes. She explained that James needed to have a heart operation. One of the valves in an artery in his heart had not closed: it usually closed later in the pregnancy than 25 weeks. His heart was getting into trouble, so the valve needed to be tied off. It was a common procedure in very premature babies, she said. James would have to be transferred to another hospital where they would make an incision under his left shoulder blade and spread the ribs. They would then insert a metal clamp.

I imagined James's tiny body, the size of an orange, being sliced open. Hot tears began to slide down my cheeks. The doctor continued to explain more and more details of the grisly procedure, until one of the nurses put her arms around me and led me away. Thankfully I never saw that doctor again.

Years later, James had to have an X-ray and the metal clamp showed up large and clear on the screen. 'He's had surgery?' asked the radiographer. 'No', I felt like saying, 'I've no idea what that is!'

The day before his operation was due to take place was 11 August 1999, the date of the first total solar eclipse visible from the UK since 1927. Most of the population stopped what they were doing and stood outside with paper masks to protect their eyes while they watched.

James was the only patient in intensive care at that time, and I had no intention of wasting what might be my last moments with him on the eclipse. The nurses left me alone, on a promise to come and get them if any alarms went off. I sat talking to James in his incubator, as a great shadow engulfed us both and then passed.

James was on a ventilator for six weeks in total. During this time the tube was taken out of his throat every now and then, and he was given 20 minutes on a device called

CPAP (continuous positive airway pressure). This involved putting a mask over his face and blowing air under pressure into his nostrils. It was designed to try to wean him off the ventilator. It was far larger and more complicated than an oxygen mask, and made him look like a Dalek. James hated it passionately. It was through his rejection of CPAP that we began to know his character. He wriggled vigorously and cried, desperately trying to prise the mask off with his minute hand.

He was, according to the nurses who saw the premature babies every day, a real fighter. The question came into our minds all the time, 'Will he live?' One day, when Andrew was visiting, he asked Dr B. 'Well,' said Dr B, 'if you pin me up against a wall I would say yes, he will live.' Dr B was just as direct when I asked for more details about how the brain damage would affect James. He sat with me and drew a chart showing three groups, representing the premature babies who had brain damage, but who were part of the 50 per cent that lived. One group at the top of his chart had few or no difficulties. The middle group, the largest, had moderate to significant difficulties. The third group at the bottom had severe difficulties, finishing with those in a persistent vegetative state. I asked Dr B where James fell. 'I can't say', he replied. 'It isn't possible to tell from a scan of people's brains exactly how they will be affected by brain damage.' He told me of a test that had once been done on a group of eminent surgeons, many of whom turned out to have abnormal brain scans!

I pressed Dr B again. He said he thought the picture would become clearer as James grew up. At present he could see that the right side of the brain was almost totally destroyed. There was some damage to the left. As the right side of the brain controls the left side of the body, it was therefore very likely that James would at least have movement difficulties down this side.

I looked at the chart and smiled. Dr B looked at me and

frowned in response. 'You are looking at this group' he said, pointing to the small group at the top of the chart with moderate or no difficulties. 'No,' I replied. 'I am looking at this.' I pointed to the largest group with moderate to significant difficulties. 'James is most likely to fall into this group. I am looking at this.' In my mind James could be quite good. And he might not be too bad.

*

I had to register his birth. It was a surreal process, as I still didn't feel that he had been born. Although he was nearly three weeks old, his due date wasn't until mid-November – another three months away. I also had to queue up in a busy registry office full of waiting people, at the time I would normally have been with James. I felt the precious minutes slipping away, and for the first time in my life I asked those around me if I could jump the queue. The response was instant acquiescence.

Over the years I gradually realised that most people think that having a disabled child is about as bad as anything they can imagine, so few will argue with your need for preferential treatment. But all that changes where money is involved, as future dealings with the Council were to show.

The birth certificate, when I got it, helped. There was his name, in black and white, 'JAMES ANDREW RACA, Date of Birth 4 August 1999' followed by an official signature. I noticed that in the days that followed, the ambiguous status I had perceived him to have – somehow only 'half born' – quietly disappeared from my mind.

In his third week we were able to give him his first bath, in a washing up bowl. It was very strange to hold his tiny arms and legs while supporting his abdomen, which was round like a ball. James was bemused and exhausted by the experience, and when returned to the familiar cocoon of his incubator, he went to sleep for the rest of the day.

Holding him was moving, as it was wonderful to have access to him. But he was so light that you could hardly feel his weight over the blankets. The sheer fragility of his body and his life was more evident than ever.

Each day in the intensive care unit felt like an aeon, so after three weeks when James had lived I began to relax a little. I drew comfort from my daily routine of visiting him and doing everything I could to be part of his life inside his plastic box. But such complacency was to be temporary.

One morning I came into the hospital to be met by a waiting nurse. I knew immediately that this meant there was a problem. When James was stable, I would simply wander in and start doing his cares. When there was an issue, I would find a consultant or lead nurse hovering, looking to grab me before I reached the incubator. The staff cared so much for the babies that their emotions formed part of the fabric of the ward. When a baby was in crisis, the air was thick with anxiety and concentration. If a baby died (and three died while James was there), the ward was silent and heavy with grief. When all the babies were stable, the nurses joked and ate biscuits and chatted with me.

Over the previous few days, the nurses had recorded James having what they described as 'cycling' movements. They had told me about this and explained that as the blood clot from the bleed in his brain dissipated, it was not unusual. However, the episodes had become more frequent and the doctor had started to give him anti-fitting medication.

On this day I was told that he had been fitting uncontrollably since the early hours. They had tried all the drugs they could think of but they couldn't stop it. In the end they had had to administer a paralysing drug to protect James from the effect of the constant seizures. The name of the drug was Paraldehyde, but I remembered it as Paraquat, which is a fatal poison. It was an appropriate name, as when

I finally saw James, he looked as dead as I could imagine. He was completely inert. Only the monitors showed he was still alive. I later discovered that Dr B had written in James's medical notes, 'The crystal ball is cloudy.'

The gravity of the nurses' faces made me realise this was very serious, and I asked to see a consultant. It was a weekend so the ward was quiet, with fewer and different staff.

I sat down in the consultant's office and was offered a cup of tea. I came to learn that in addition to finding staff waiting for me, this too was an ominous sign. The nurses didn't usually have the time to make cups of tea for parents. I didn't think I had seen this consultant before. She had curly brown hair, a wide mouth and a kind face.

She told me gently that if the fitting didn't stop within the next five to seven days it would mean that James's brain was so irreparably damaged that there would have to be a decision on whether to turn off his life support. It would not be a decision Andrew and I could take on our own, nor could the doctors take it alone: we would all have to reach it together.

I couldn't stay in the hospital. I could hardly drive and barely speak as I arrived home. Andrew was at work, and I don't even remember when I told him and what happened when I did. We were immersed in our own private worlds of grief. Years later, I found out that his boss was not being as supportive as Andrew would have expected. He thought the boss was feeling vulnerable at work, and if Andrew left there would be 'one less mouth to feed'. He was taking advantage of Andrew's lack of concentration to edge him out of the company. In his state of shock and disorientation, Andrew felt the one contribution he could make to our situation was to try to hold on to his job, by turning up at the office.

The next day I had to take Tom to buy some new shoes (he had none that fitted) and go to the supermarket (we had no food). Tom and shoes did not go well together. There was a long queue in the shoe shop and I was trying to deal with a stressed two-year-old who was making the most of a rare few hours with his Mummy. I felt like saying to the staff and the waiting customers 'Excuse me, my baby may die in the next few days, do you think I could go first?' But so great was my terror that I couldn't bear to hear myself saying it. When we got to the supermarket, I couldn't even choose between the frozen pizzas, and after ten minutes I left with nothing.

The next day was a Monday and Tom was back at nursery. I had not heard from the hospital so I was holding my breath. As I drove into the car park outside the neonatal unit I saw Karen. She had not been around at the weekend when I saw the unknown consultant, but she knew James was very ill. She explained that I would not be seeing her for the next month as she was off to visit her mother in Malaysia. I felt as if I was losing Karen at the worst possible time, and it must have shown on my face. Then she took me by the shoulders. 'Look Jane,' she said, 'I know how much you love James. But sometimes, if someone's very badly damaged, it's better to let them go. My mother is paralysed. She can't do anything. I save up all my leave and go home to nurse her for one month each year. If you lose James now it'll be very painful for a while, but then you'll move on with your life.' I heard what she said but it was meaningless to me. I couldn't lose my son.

As I approached the unit I almost walked in with my eyes shut rather than risk seeing a waiting presence. But the small glass window in the door to intensive care was empty. No one was looking out for me, and I approached James's incubator alone.

He was no longer inert and I saw a little dark pool of one eye gazing at me through a slit in his drowsy eyelids. For once, I didn't ask any questions but just began to do his cares. I didn't ask any questions for the next seven days and no one said anything. It was as if the conversation at the weekend with the unknown consultant had never happened. It took two weeks before I could bring myself to ask whether James was still on anti-fitting medication, and then I was told that he had been off it for some time.

One Sunday when the ward was quiet, I caught the consultant on duty in her office. This time it was Dr A, whom I had met a couple of times before. Emboldened by James's continued survival, and the diagram from Dr B which had shown that James might be 'quite good', I asked if we could have a little chat. I wanted to know what James might be like, what the future might hold. The nurse went to get me a cup of tea, an ominous sign which I missed.

I now realise that Dr A was very restrained in what she said, which was wise, as I didn't last very long. Dr B had spoken in generalities. Dr A started talking about cerebral palsy, which she said people used to call 'spastic', and about how James would wear callipers – now called splints – and special shoes.

Vivid images of my school days in the 1960s and 1970s came into my thoughts. A boy with metal callipers and a large ugly black platform shoe. I remembered the word 'spastic' as an insult. 'They make very nice shoes now' said Dr A, as if reading my thoughts. 'Little blue ones that look like sports shoes.' But my face was awash and I had to leave the hospital.

One day I arrived to be met by nurses waving at me and cheering. James had been weaned off the ventilator and CPAP, which he had tolerated from time to time, and was breathing only with the help of an oxygen mask. He had made the permanent transition from intensive care to the high dependency ward. Now I could hold him without having to be careful that I didn't knock the ventilator, and I could breast-feed him, provided I had a handy pipe to waft oxygen over his nostrils.

At first he could only take a couple of sucks before getting very tired. But it was deeply moving to see his heart rate slow as he relaxed into being held and then drifted off to sleep – to see the physical effects of food and love at work.

Tom was able to come in now and see James and to understand better where Mummy had been disappearing to for so many weeks. This family time had been delayed for unbearably long, and had looked on more than one occasion as if it would slip away altogether.

Tom had had to cope with a massive upheaval to his life. Having been cared for at home for two years, he was suddenly thrust full time into nursery, and when he returned he had all of the emotions and talk of hospitals swirling around. One night I was reading him a bedtime story called *The Baby Who Wouldn't Go to Bed*.[2] In it, the naughty baby gets into his toy car and goes off on adventures, instead of going to sleep. But as he gets further and further from home, darkness falls and he becomes frightened. Then his Mummy comes to find him and carries him home to bed. I thought of James being away from me for so much of the time, and that I couldn't carry him home. My voice began to get thick with emotion. Then, with that intuition which small children sometimes display and which takes your breath away, Tom closed the book and suggested we find another story.

The battle for James's life may have been over, but the battle for his long-term health was just beginning. No one knew how well he could really see or hear. A consultant ophthalmologist had checked his vision and explained that the blood vessels at the back of James's eyes had not finished developing when he was born and were going astray. The high levels of oxygen he was receiving made it worse. The condition, retinopathy of prematurity, had various levels of severity. At the moment, in his left eye it was at stage three. If it reached stage four it would mean the retina was partially detached and James would lose part or all of his sight in that eye. There was nothing anyone could do except wait and watch.

   2 *The Baby Who Wouldn't Go to Bed by Helen Cooper,
published by Corgi Children's books 2007.*

Every so often I would arrive to find James had big red circles around his eyes where the eye consultant had pressed the circular glass that she used to keep his eyes open while she looked into them.

One day I was getting a nappy when the nurse came up to me. 'There is a doctor who wants to look at James's eyes', she said. 'I have told him he needs your permission.' I was puzzled, as I knew the eye consultant had just left. 'Is it necessary to have another examination?' I asked. She looked at me for a minute. 'He's training to be a consultant', she said. 'He should've come earlier to watch, but he was late.'

I thought of the babies the doctor could help when he had finished his training. Then I looked at James's red eyes. 'No,' I said. 'I don't give permission. He should've been here on time.'

Over those weeks I came to know the names and habits of all the nurses and consultants, and I could predict when a ward round would be late because a certain consultant was taking it. I knew that, when reporting on progress, some erred on the side of optimism and some would always leave you in despair. The junior doctors though, made less of an impression. This was partly because they were on rotation and didn't stay on the ward long, and partly because their youth and inexperience made them the least likely to be able to engage with parents. Not being parents themselves and concentrating, as they were, on the technicalities, they seemed oblivious to the acute emotions surrounding them on the ward.

When the consultants were on ward round I wasn't allowed to stay with James, in order to protect the privacy of the medical conversations about the other babies. Then I used to chat to the ward clerk, who sat just outside intensive care.

One day she told me that her desk was on the same spot as the bed on which she had lain, aged 16, when her baby was born with the cord around its neck. It had been taken away, though she was sure it could have been saved today, she said. They didn't even give it a chance.

It made the hairs prickle on my forearms to think of her sitting there, as close as she could, to the soul of her lost baby.

James was finally moved to the cot nursery when he was almost weaned off oxygen. His retinopathy had regressed and his eyes were out of danger. He spoiled things a bit by having a 'braddy' and turning blue a few days before he was due to come home. The intensive care team ran in, tickled his feet and stuck an oxygen mask on and he revived.

I would go in and find that Karen (who had returned from Malaysia) had turned the oxygen supply down a little each day, as much as James could stand. She would look at me wide eyed and make a 'shush' sign against her lips. She explained to me that if the babies heard their mothers being told that the oxygen had been turned down, then they became 'naughty' and started playing up.

Eventually all wires and tubes were off and James lay there in an open cot, freely accessible to me to be picked up and cuddled or bathed. The liberty was sweet as honey.

One baby was abandoned. I realised after a while that no one was coming to visit her. I asked the nurses and they said that she had brain damage and the family didn't want her. The nurses would all sneak in whenever they had a minute and cuddle that baby.

The babies in the cot room were able to make noises, partly because they weren't ventilated or with oxygen masks, but also because they were older. Some babies came there who had not been premature but had just had a few problems after birth and were of normal weight. With their huge chubby faces and rolls of fat on their thighs, they looked like giants compared with James.

There were a lot of Asian mums in the unit and I saw how wonderful it was for them to have support from their extended families. I heard from one Muslim mum that when she went home, she would be looked after by female family members for 40 days, giving her time to recover fully from the birth. By the time James went home it would be four months since I had given birth, but I would still have loved to spend a few weeks in bed, being cooked for and sleeping! My broken nights were just about to begin.

James came home after 100 days in hospital, weighing 5lbs. He had been born 15 weeks early, weighing 1lb 12oz. His homecoming was a strange anticlimax after so much drama, possibly because the weight of responsibility for him was now fully on me.

Chapter 3
HOLDING OUR BREATH
1999-2000

For the first few days after James came home I was very nervous. I had persuaded the hospital to let me borrow a portable monitor which would beep if James stopped breathing. Without that I wouldn't have been able to sleep at all. Gradually though, I became more and more relaxed, as the horror of the days in hospital began to recede and James seemed to be well. I finally took the monitor off when I realised that it had been beeping while he had been asleep in his cot and I had been in the garden. I hadn't even heard it. It had come unstuck from James's chest and he was fine. I realised then that I didn't need it any more.

Once I had let go of the tension of the hospital, the next few months were a time of introversion, as I sank into a domestic cocoon of carpets, central heating and silence. After all those weeks of the most intense emotional trauma, and dealing with the sheer practicality of hospital visits, it was a relief to wake up – even in the middle of the night – and to know that the following day could be spent entirely at home.

I didn't mind when James woke me in the night for a feed, because several times over the course of his hospital stay I had thought that I would never have that experience again.

Andrew and I still felt very close to the nurses on the unit, and they visited us for about ten weeks after James came home, weighing him on a little portable scale as if he were a cake.

Before James's birth I had been the chair of the local

branch of the National Childbirth Trust (NCT). Once James came home I felt able to chair a meeting at my house. That was quite an evening. One mother told us about a friend who had had an affair two months after the birth of her child, and was now pregnant as a result. We all fell silent as we contemplated feeling energetic enough eight weeks after giving birth to have sex with our usual partners, never mind anyone new. Then Andrew brought James in for a breast-feed. There was an electric silence as the smallest baby that any of us had ever seen was handed over and plugged to the breast.

At that meeting, I got to see the draft autumn edition of our NCT newsletter. In it was an article by a member who had had a baby with Down's syndrome a few months earlier. The timing of it was poignant to me, particularly as she was one of the mothers who had written to me when James was born. She had been asked to talk about her experience of giving birth. She did so like any other mother describing her labour experience. Of course, what people really wanted to know, in her situation, was what it felt like to give birth to a child who wasn't 'normal'. She dealt with that by quoting an article which is well known among parents of disabled children, 'Welcome to Holland'.

Welcome To Holland
by
Emily Perl Kingsley [3]

I am often asked to describe the experience of raising a child with a disability - to try to help people who have not shared that unique experience to understand it, to imagine how it would feel. It's like this......

When you're going to have a baby, it's like planning a fabulous vacation trip - to Italy. You buy a bunch of guide books and make your wonderful plans. The Coliseum. The Michelangelo

---

[3] *Reproduced as per the original at the request of the author.*

David. The gondolas in Venice. You may learn some handy phrases in Italian. It's all very exciting.

After months of eager anticipation, the day finally arrives. You pack your bags and off you go. Several hours later, the plane lands. The flight attendant comes in and says, "Welcome to Holland."

"Holland?!?" you say. "What do you mean Holland?? I signed up for Italy! I'm supposed to be in Italy. All my life I've dreamed of going to Italy."

But there's been a change in the flight plan. They've landed in Holland and there you must stay.

The important thing is that they haven't taken you to a horrible, disgusting, filthy place, full of pestilence, famine and disease. It's just a different place.

So you must go out and buy new guide books. And you must learn a whole new language. And you will meet a whole new group of people you would never have met.

It's just a different place. It's slower-paced than Italy, less flashy than Italy. But after you've been there for a while and you catch your breath, you look around.... and you begin to notice that Holland has windmills....and Holland has tulips. Holland even has Rembrandts.

But everyone you know is busy coming and going from Italy... and they're all bragging about what a wonderful time they had there. And for the rest of your life, you will say "Yes, that's where I was supposed to go. That's what I had planned."

And the pain of that will never, ever, ever, ever go away... because the loss of that dream is a very very significant loss.

But... if you spend your life mourning the fact that you didn't get to Italy, you may never be free to enjoy the very special, the very lovely things ... about Holland.

©1987 by Emily Perl Kingsley. All rights reserved.
Reprinted by permission of the author.

*

As it was now late November, I put James in a turquoise Eskimo suit when we went out. It was the smallest I could find but was still vastly too big for him. The arms and legs of the suit extended far beyond James's hands and feet, so he looked like a little starfish. I later heard from women who became close friends, that they had an image of me walking along the path to Tom's school, clutching this tiny star-like figure, looking as if I had the world on my shoulders.

In early December, we had our first visit from a physiotherapist. It was to be the first of many home visits to monitor James's physical progress. He had a tendency to lie on his right, and his head was so soft that it had become flat on that side. It was most disconcerting to look at him, as he resembled a claw hammer.

On the physiotherapist's advice I went to the market and bought a sausage-shaped draft excluder, embroidered as a snake. I wound it into an orange and green scaly coil, and rested James's head in it, like a macabre nest. It prevented him from lying on his side, which made me feel very mean, but within a week the shape of his head was becoming more spherical.

I said to the physiotherapist how useful it was to have her come to the house. She told me that the physiotherapy service in our area didn't have the resources to provide therapy to all the children who needed it. So they concentrated their efforts on the younger children with whom they could make the biggest difference. I remember

45

feeling naively astonished that in this country, resources for physically disabled children could be so limited.

We had two months of respite from trauma, and then James became ill. We had been brave enough to travel 100 miles south to stay with my family in Surrey for Christmas. I so yearned to be normal again that when I thought I saw a bluish tinge to James's skin, as he sat enveloped in his car seat, I ignored it and carried on driving. Over the next few days, he developed an ominous cough, and with growing unease we came home early. We rang the nurses on the neonatal unit and were genuinely shocked to find that he could no longer be admitted there but had to go to the general children's ward, via A&E.

He had bronchiolitis, a virus affecting the tiny blood vessels in the lungs. It made him struggle to breathe and there was no cure other than to support him in fighting the infection. He was too weak to feed so he was put on a drip. A large plastic box was put over his head into which, I was told, warm humidified air would be pumped. It took a long time to set this up and by the time air began to flow into the box it was 2am. I had been trying and failing to feed a hungry James the whole of the previous night and my eyelids were shutting against my will. It would have been so easy to collapse onto the camp bed set up for me on the floor next to James's cot. Just a bit longer, I told myself, until the warm air comes through.

The air came through, but it was cold and damp, not warm and humid. I called the nurse. She was irritated, as the ward was very busy. She told me the air would get warm soon and left. I watched the cold air gradually fill James's infected lungs, so recently struggling to come off oxygen.

I couldn't stand it and called her back. I made her feel the air. She waved her hand inside the box. 'It's meant to be like that' she said, and left again. I could feel the tears of exhaustion and despair welling up. Then I saw a phone on the wall with a list of ward numbers next to it. There at the bottom was the neonatal unit. I picked up the phone and dialled. Karen answered. 'Is the air in the head box supposed to be cold?' I asked, so low in spirits that I doubted my own reason. 'No', she said, shocked.

I begged her to come to the ward but of course she couldn't. Never mind, I had an ally now. I called the irritable nurse again. I told her what Karen had said and she took the head box away and brought another one. Later she at least had the grace to come in and tell me that the first one was broken. Not all parents stayed with their children on the ward overnight. I wondered what would have happened to James if I hadn't been there.

He was discharged on 31 December 1999. That night I sat feeding him in his bedroom while the fireworks boomed and blazed, lighting up the sky outside the window, welcoming in the new Millennium. There was no celebration I could have gone to that would have bettered the one I was sharing with my younger son.

*

The year 2000 fell sharply into two halves. For the first six months we continued to revel in James being alive, as did our family and friends. We hadn't told our friends yet about the brain damage. We still hoped that having survived against the odds, James might yet prove to have the most minimal of difficulties. Perhaps, like another child we knew, he would just have a weakness down one side and difficulty in tying his shoelaces. We were not in the game of speculating. The whole issue of disability was in a big dark box which we didn't need to open yet. With breathtaking insensitivity, some people tried to do it for us.

'Is he, y'know, *alright*?' said one. 'Has he suffered any brain damage?' asked another breezily, as if she were enquiring whether he liked spaghetti. Both were met with a bright smile and a false affirmation that James was indeed unscathed by his early birth. The pain those questions caused though, before we were ready for them, was exquisite.

There was, as yet, no sign of the effects of the brain damage, and he appeared to be a normal baby. The wrinkled red frog had disappeared, to be replaced by a prince, with even features, large blue eyes and very blond hair. He was interested in people, gazing into their eyes and smiling when they approached. Strangers would stop me in the street to tell me how handsome he was and to hold his hand. This was bittersweet, as I wondered how they would feel about him if they knew the truth.

He looked much younger than he was, due to his small size and the delayed development he was 'allowed' to have, on account of having been so ill for so long. He didn't babble, and wasn't very bendy. He didn't grab his toes and suck them, like other babies. I was told this was because he had lain flat in his incubator for so many weeks rather than curled up in the womb. However, at the first follow-up appointments, no one could detect either genuine developmental delay, or signs of cerebral palsy. Dr B wrote:

'He is smiling and I cannot detect signs of cerebral palsy yet. We are of course looking for it on the left side of the body more than the right, and maybe it will be more in evidence when he sees Dr. A in a month's time. I plan to review him again in May, but at the moment, I am more optimistic about James than I have ever been.'

We were holding our breath.

James was still vulnerable to chest problems and I spent several more nights next to him on the children's ward. I became quite blasé about it, a bit of a camp-bed veteran.

He continued to see the eye consultant, who diagnosed him as having a squint which would require glasses.

Going to the eye hospital was an eye-opener. The

environment was designed for blind or partially-sighted people. There were enormous Braille buttons in the lift, which also spoke with a posh woman's voice telling you whether you were going up or down and to which floor. There were handrails everywhere, to help feel your way around. The toys in the children's play area were unusually robust, with an emphasis on very shiny and colourful patterns.

When James was examined, the ophthalmologist would shine a torch in his eyes and then try to make him look this way and that by wiggling a soft toy. James was much more interested in the ophthalmologist's face than the toys, and it seemed to me that he was impossible to test in this way.

Sometimes he would get to see the consultant, who would use the dreaded glass discs. He would observe her with a steady gaze, with what we described as his 'Winston Churchill' look, as if daring her to go ahead. I noticed that the consultant engaged with us better when Andrew was present than when I was on my own. He attended appointments in his business suit and made a tall and impressive figure. I had lost interest in my appearance and lived in leggings and sweatshirts, a situation which was to continue for a long time.

The turning point in the year came when James was officially diagnosed with cerebral palsy.

Dr A had begun to comment to me, when she bent his legs and arms gently to the left and right, that she detected stiffness in his left side. I wasn't surprised, as I had been expecting it since he was born. In July Andrew came with me to see her. Dr A was more grave than usual and said that she felt she could now say with certainty that James had spastic cerebral palsy. She explained that this meant that there was nothing actually wrong with his arms and legs, but the brain damage meant that the electrical signals from his brain to his limbs were distorted. They were making the muscles contract, which in turn made his limbs stiff.

I was quite relieved to have the issue of his disability

out in the open. I had lived with the physical reality of James all day every day, sometimes all night too, for nearly a year. I had become ready to share the news about his brain damage with our friends and was finding it difficult to keep it to myself. Andrew, however, had kept putting it off. He was only able to dip in and out of this world and was less prepared for it than I was. His voice was thick with tears as he shook Dr A's hand and said 'One day, James will stand up and be counted.' 'I'm sure he will,' replied Dr A, with quiet conviction.

There is a lot of power in a label. Once James was officially diagnosed as having cerebral palsy, things started to happen. I didn't realise it then, but a pathway lay ahead of him which the health professionals were all familiar with, but which was invisible to me.

The first sign was an increase in home visits by the physiotherapist and a referral to the hearing service.

I was not concerned about his hearing. I had spent too many nights creeping past his room, trying not to wake him and failing, to be in any doubt that his ears were functioning perfectly.

Nevertheless, we had some amusing visits to the hospital, involving more furry toys. They carried out what I called the 'pink pig test'. I would sit with James on my lap in a soundproof room. On each side of the room was a fluffy pink mechanical pig. One of the pigs would start to snuffle and oink. If James turned to the pig it was supposed to show he could hear. He would find the pigs hysterically funny. He sat on my knee shaking with laughter at the sight of them until I joined in too.

By now I was beginning to realise he had a cheeky sense of humour. When I was changing him, no sooner would I have done up one side of his nappy and moved to the other than he would give a wicked chuckle, hold my gaze and deliberately undo the first tab. This was very uplifting because it showed he was aware and alert. Despite the cerebral palsy there was still no obvious developmental delay, and Dr B was saying that James fell within the normal range of cognitive ability for his age. Following standard practice, he treated James as having been born on his due date rather than his actual birthday. This gave James an 'adjusted age', to take into account his four months in an incubator.

We began, tentatively, to tell people about the diagnosis. We experimented with different forms of wording. We found it best to say simply that James had been diagnosed with cerebral palsy, because most people didn't know what that was, and so it gave us the opportunity to explain. We learned to avoid using the words 'brain damage' at all costs, particularly with people who had not met James, as it seemed to conjure up alarming pictures of a bedridden victim, when the boy we were getting to know was far from that.

Gradually, the words started to come out pat, although we could never be prepared for the reactions we got. Some people became quite interested, and started asking for details of the prognosis. 'Will he walk?' they asked, 'Will he be affected mentally?'

Fielding such questions when we had no answers was intensely draining, and made some days unbearable. We came to appreciate the kindness and wisdom of those who just remained silent. Most of our good friends seemed unsurprised. Helen, my lawyer friend, just said 'So, what do you call him, Jane – James or Jamie?' 'Well,' I said, 'we usually call him Jamesy Wamesy Woobedy Doobedy, but Jamie will do.'

*

In August James was one, and we came up against the mixed emotions involved in celebrating the birth of a disabled child.

The day of James's birth was the worst of my life, and I didn't want to remember it at all. James was too young to understand or appreciate his birthday, so it went unmarked. I later met other parents of disabled children who felt this paradox. Of course they loved their children and wanted to celebrate them. But the actual anniversary of the child's birth brought back all the pain of dashed expectations as the parents realised, either at birth or later, that the child they had been expecting was not the child they had.

I did take a cake to the neonatal unit though, saying 'James Raca was one on 4 August 2000, thank-you for his life.' Karen told me off for spending so much money, although I could see she was pleased. She said she would hide it from the junior doctors as none of them had looked after James and they would eat in it a trice. I agreed that the cake belonged to the nurses.

On the way back from the hospital I spotted the new vicar's wife from our local parish walking down the road with a baby who looked a similar age to James. I pulled over for a chat and she invited me in for a cup of tea. She was a tiny, pretty woman who looked very tired. She was called Joanna and she explained that she had five children, of whom her baby son, Edmund, was the youngest. Then she told me something that would make her one of the most important friends I ever had. She told me that Edmund was autistic.

I didn't know much about autism then, except that I had seen the film *Rain Man* in the 1980s.

I noticed that Edmund didn't babble or make eye contact or smile. James lay on the mat in front of the fireplace, gazed at Joanna and beamed happily. Edmund was silent and preoccupied. 'James is very smiley', she said. 'I am so envious. It's hard to have a child who doesn't "give back" in the normal way.' I told her that I was envious that Edmund could crawl.

We talked about the moment when we had had our respective diagnoses. I told her we had known since birth that James had brain damage. She told me that she and the vicar had thought Edmund was normal until they realised he was not passing the usual developmental milestones. I could see that it was a cause of great pain to her, and it occurred to me that in a strange way Andrew and I were lucky. We were prepared for the worst from the beginning. We had been spared the shock of thinking for any length of time that we had a normal baby, only to find out later that he was disabled.

Joanna went on to tell me of a friend who had popped round when she heard Edmund was autistic. The friend also had an autistic son, but hers was much older than Ed. As she had come into the vicarage she had left him in the car, which had been rocking and bucking in the road. 'I daren't bring him in' said the friend; 'he's not in a good mood today.' Joanna had looked at Edmund and wondered what on earth lay in store.

In October, James had his first pair of glasses. They stayed on his head for about three seconds and then were pulled off disdainfully. This was the beginning of a two-year battle which would eventually have me tying James's sleeves together, straitjacket style, to stop him reaching the glasses. The consultant had said that there was a window of opportunity to correct vision up until the age of seven, when a child's eyes were fully formed. I absolutely must get James to wear the glasses.

The stress of trying was crushing. I had special curly bits put on to the end of the sides to go round James's ears, so the glasses stayed on. It made no difference. The glasses were repeatedly bitten, chewed, thrown, smashed, and discarded. I was back at the opticians every two weeks getting a new pair. I felt such a failure that I began to lie to the ophthalmologist about how much time James was spending with them on. Once or twice I tried tentatively to explain the difficulty. But I felt so guilty about being unable to get on top of the situation that I found it hard to say 'There is no way I can get this child to keep the glasses on.' The ophthalmologist was sympathetic but could only reiterate that we had a short window of opportunity before James's sight was set forever. No pressure there then.

By December, Andrew and I were desperate for a real break. We had James and Tom with us all the time and no one to look after them, even for a night, since it would be too much to ask the people we knew to take responsibility for James. It didn't occur to us that we might be entitled to some help. We felt that we couldn't leave the children anywhere, but we thought we could at least get a meaningful change of scene by going abroad.

We had not felt brave enough to go very far since James had been born, but he had been pretty healthy all year, with no more hospital episodes since the previous Christmas. The idea of a holiday was overwhelmingly seductive.

We ruled out any destination which was more than a three-hour flight away and consulted Dr B as to which places had reliable hospitals. We picked on a hotel in Cyprus which had a crèche for Tom, and we imagined child-free evenings and quiet days swimming in the hotel pool.

The reality was that we managed to snatch two days of weak sunshine before James turned blue and started coughing. He had bronchiolitis again, so I spent Christmas with him in a Greek hospital, while Andrew and Tom were left at the hotel.

The brief high we had felt on arriving in blue skies – that sense of the excitement of a normal family holiday, so very sweet after such abstinence – came crashing to the ground like the end of a sugar rush. We could not get away from James's condition, his vulnerability. The idea that we could escape had been an illusion.

A cold dark feeling lodged in part of my heart and never quite went away.

While I was in the Greek hospital I met a gentle handsome doctor who told me of a therapy which he had personally seen could significantly improve function in spastic limbs. It involved putting the child inside an oxygen chamber and giving him (or her) pressurised air, like a diver with the bends. The theory was that this saturated the blood with oxygen and helped restore areas of the brain which had been damaged. The doctor urged me to get James treated when I returned to England. I looked into his big dark eyes and promised.

The experience of having James ill abroad was so terrifying that it was two and a half years until we set foot outside England again. Kind friends tried to persuade us that they could cope with having James along. Surely we would like to share their villa in the south of France, or Italy, there was plenty of space?

We would hesitate for a moment, while visions of heat, wine and olives would dance in our heads, then with great wistfulness we would decline to join them.

*

In 2000 we had a total of ten hospital appointments and two emergency admissions.

Chapter 4
HIS PLACE ON THE CHART
2001

In 2001 I began taking James to a music class for toddlers. I had noticed that he became excited by music and would rock vigorously whenever we played anything, particularly pop, on the CD player. Although he couldn't crawl, he looked like any other child of his age, and I wanted to do normal things with him, as I had done with Tom. I hadn't taken James out into that world before though. All of our outings had been to hospitals or with close friends - people who knew and understood. This was a public group of mothers with their own offspring to think about.

The teacher was very sympathetic and took care to slow down the music for 'Head, shoulders, knees and toes'. I was then able to help James slowly reach the various bits of his body, which the other children did oh so quickly.

We were made very welcome at first. However, after a few weeks even that benign environment began to feel hostile. There was a mother there who felt as if she had to protect her son from James. On one occasion she placed an arm between him and her child, while we were all sitting in a circle on the floor. When I looked at her questioningly, she gave me a rictus smile.

When we put our instruments away at the end of a percussion session, I would help James to take his maracas and put them in the tub. But I had to support him and move his legs and arms. The room would fall silent as I did so, and I felt uncomfortable.

We stopped going to that music class after a few months and, in the spring, I started taking James to Pram Pushers, the local toddler group I had attended with Tom. They were still singing nursery rhymes like 'Wind the bobbin up' and 'He's a dingle dangle scarecrow with a flippy floppy hat', which I remembered from my own childhood. But those Monday morning sessions with James were very different from taking Tom. Although I knew the group leader well, and some of the other mums, I felt apart from them in a way I hadn't before. Then I had been able to share cups of bitter instant coffee and chat about broken nights and temper tantrums. Now I couldn't leave James for a second in case the other children trod on him; he also needed my left hand in order to play with the toys.

At break time all the children sat on the floor around low tables eating crisps and bits of apple. James couldn't sit up and had to lean forward on his elbows, like someone prostrating himself in prayer. He was able to pull up a bit though, in order to eat his favourite food, crisps. Once his crisps were gone he didn't hesitate to start eating other children's. I wasn't quite sure how to react when he did this and neither were the other mothers. I knew he shouldn't do it, but I was so delighted to see him with other children in a normal setting that I didn't want to upset him. The other mothers didn't want to get cross with a disabled child. So there was a lot of whispering between mums and their normal offspring about 'sharing nicely'.

One mum was a young GP. She had the medical background to be professionally interested in James, but not the wisdom and experience to manage it. 'When was he born?' she asked. 'At 25 weeks' I replied. She thought for a moment as she recollected her medical training. Then her expression brightened. 'Oh, that's OK', she said. 'Twenty-five weeks is OK.' I thought about James's four months in the neonatal unit and his damaged brain. Twenty-five weeks definitely wasn't all right, it wasn't all right at all. But this wasn't an argument I was going to have with her, in front of all the children.

*

My mind kept returning to the Greek doctor from our Cyprus holiday. His dark eyes may have swayed me temporarily, but the thought that James might be partially cured by the oxygen therapy had put me on an unstoppable quest. I started researching places that offered it. It didn't seem to be available on the NHS and wasn't easy to find. I eventually came across a charity which was advertising its oxygen tanks. I wrote to Dr B, James's consultant from the neonatal unit, and he was sceptical about it.

'My heart sinks when parents present me with alternative therapies to help their child who is at risk of disability. What parents would not sell all their possessions to give their child a chance of normality? My general approach to unproven therapies is to accept them if they cost nothing, do no harm and don't put the family through a great deal of stress. Evening primrose oil and reflexology spring to mind... I am sorry if I sound cynical and but [sic] I will accept treatment only if it is subjected to proper trials in real journals.'

I should have been cautious, but I felt I just had to give the oxygen therapy a chance. I went to visit the charity with Katherine, a GP friend from London. However when we arrived we were told that the oxygen was now rarely used, because other techniques were proving more successful. These included the taking of supplements and a form of physical therapy which seemed to consist of tapping the patient for periods of time each day. The tapping technique was taught to parents and carers, who returned at intervals for supervised sessions costing £50 per hour. No proper medical history was taken – we just completed a short form with James's diagnosis.

I was upset to find that the oxygen therapy, which I had asked about in advance, was not being used.

The supplements person was not there. I was sceptical about the tapping therapy. The response to my scepticism was to demonstrate it on me. I had the pleasure of an enthusiastic tapping session by a male member of staff.

I finally walked out in tears of rage, clutching a prescription for James of £9,500 worth of treatment, including oxygen therapy and supplements.

I should have listened to Dr B. That was the end of alternative treatments for me. I gave up on the oxygen tanks, even though I had never tried them.

I had also heard about another more mainstream form of therapy, called conductive education. The National Institute of Conductive Education was only two miles from our home, and based its approach on the Peto Institute in Hungary, which I had heard of. I decided to give it a go.

The headquarters was based in a stately building in beautiful grounds on the edge of a park. The first time I visited it I was overwhelmed. The place was full of disabled children, some in wheelchairs, some walking in unfamiliar postures. All were moving with determination.

They were being alternately teased and encouraged by the instructors, who were mostly from Hungary. 'Chloe put your foot up, what is it doing down there, has it gone to sleep? It is not night time yet, could you have a word with it?' The place had a legitimacy which the other charity had lacked. It had a reception desk, secretaries, and a proper assessment process. It also had an atmosphere of optimism and excitement - so unlike the desperation I had sensed in the other place.

The philosophy here was to help disabled children to move around in the normal world, using normal equipment. So they would sit on ordinary chairs at ordinary tables for lunch, and use ordinary toilets. It felt to me like a place where the disabled world and the normal world came together, and I was comfortable there. James and I started attending parent and child classes twice each week and carried on until he was three.

There were only a few other families in his class, so once the ice was broken we found out a little of each other's histories. Lawrence's mother had been in labour for too long, and he had been starved of oxygen at birth. His limbs were floppy rather than stiff. He couldn't sit or even support the weight of his own head. When he ate, the muscles in his throat couldn't direct the food properly and some ended up in his lungs. His mother eventually opted for a gastrostomy, where a tube was placed directly through his abdomen into his stomach, with a valve on the outside. In this way she could feed him directly without the danger of him choking. She still gave him the odd chocolate button at snack time though, which melted in his mouth and stopped him feeling left out.

Rachel had Rett syndrome, which meant that her skills peaked at the age of two and then she regressed. Her hands were constantly moving and she had difficulty holding objects such as spoons and toys. I was reminded of Joanna's son, Edmund. I thought how awful it would be to believe you had a normal child, and then to realise they were not developing as you expected, or worse, that they were losing the skills they already had.

We began to compare our predicaments. Rachel's mum Fiona and I thought Lawrence's mother was lucky, because although Lawrence was floppy, he was bright. He helped to decorate the Christmas tree by pointing with his eyes where the baubles should be hung. Rachel's mother envied me James's happy nature. It was true that he was a laughing cavalier, but his concentration span was a nanosecond, and if you sat him up he would gradually lean over, like the Tower of Pisa. Rachel could sit up and walk, at least for the time being.

Parents of non-disabled children overhearing these conversations would probably have thought them rather sick. To us they seemed natural and infinitely preferable to benchmarking our children against their mainstream contemporaries. Like so much flotsam and jetsam on a beach with a retreating tide, our children were being left inexorably behind.

*

James still wasn't speaking and he was now 18 months old. I wrote to Dr A, who was going to be James's consultant on an ongoing basis, to monitor his development. (He was still seeing Dr B as a former neonate, but this would not continue.) I had accepted that James would have some physical difficulties and maybe learning difficulties, but I had never contemplated that he might not speak any words at all. I asked Dr A if the weeks spent with a ventilator down his throat might have damaged his vocal chords. My letter to her was a classic exercise in denial.

She didn't respond by telling me that he probably would never speak, which I am sure she must have suspected. Instead she referred him to the local child development centre, a place which would take us a long way down the invisible path which the professionals could see and we couldn't. Here they would assess his entire development, with a raft of therapists.

But before James could get to the child development centre, Dr B was able to place him on the chart he had first drawn for me in the neonatal unit. It was the one dividing the premature babies who survived into three ability groups. This time it was I, not Andrew, who asked Dr B to take a guess at the future and say what he thought the outcome was for James. The answer was that he was in the middle of the spectrum. Dr B's letter to the GP following our appointment said:

61

'I note James is not yet speaking and although he is a pleasant smiley baby he does not strike me as a child who is developmentally normal from an intellectual point of view. Mother asked me what I felt my gut feeling was about him.... At first I avoided committing myself, as of course this is an area where there is great capacity for recovery. However, when pinned to the wall, I told her my gut feeling was that James would not make normal school. She was understandably upset but by the end of the consultation I think she felt she agreed with me. I think my role with James is now over. I will leave his follow up to Dr [A].'

James would have to go to a special school. He wasn't at the bottom of the chart which Dr B had drawn for me in the neonatal unit, but neither was he near the top, which is what I had begun to dare to hope.

The next few months were searingly painful, as James was assessed by one health professional after another, and his difficulties and delays were catalogued.

We were used to the physiotherapist coming to the house and giving me tasks to do with James. I had to massage the ball at the base of his left thumb twice a day, to loosen its vice-like attachment to his fingers. However, to her visits were added those of the speech therapist, who asked me to mouth words in an exaggerated way when I spoke, so that James could see my lips. She also asked me to make sure I offered James choices in what he ate, drank or played with.

Then came the visiting teacher who wanted me to have a play session a day where I helped James to post objects or turn knobs. He couldn't use his left hand at all so he needed mine to be placed over his. Finally there was the occupational therapist who asked me to make sure James had time out of his high chair or pushchair so he could get sensory input. 'Some messy play would be good as well' she said. 'Try cornflour and water gloop.'

By the time all of these people had seen enough of James

to write their reports, I had begun to resent them bitterly. My day was now divided into micro tasks which centred entirely on James. Interwoven with these were hospital appointments, visits to the optician to get James's glasses mended yet again, and sessions of conductive education. I just about managed to feed and clothe us all (me in leggings) but Tom was being ominously neglected. He was now four and able to start telling us meaningfully how awful things were for him.

One weekend he startled us by blurting out that he must be the loneliest boy in the world. He had never articulated any emotion in such a way before and I remember feeling cold and sick when I heard that. It has left me with a permanent burden of guilt about him. Even though James doesn't live with us now, I still feel I can never do enough for Tom, to make up for the years when we couldn't give him what he needed.

I try to forgive myself, as when I look back on it we had a child who wasn't walking or talking but who showed some signs of being able to do so. We were being told by all the therapists that the greatest difference could be made at an early age, and they encouraged us to put endless therapies into practice to achieve this. It wasn't a conscious decision, but what parents in our situation would spend their energy taking their able child to music lessons and football practice rather than teach the disabled one how to move and speak? That is the reality we faced.

Yet we did have the balance wrong, and I resolved to do something about it. I got in touch with yet another charity to see if they could provide a specialist carer to look after James when Tom came home from school, so I could spend some time with my neglected older son.

So carers came and then they went. There was one enormous woman who sat on the floor enveloping James in acres of bosom while they watched videos together. Then she disappeared, never to return. There was a hysterical woman with very long hair, who just wanted to talk about her sister, who was having a nervous breakdown and painting the glass on her windows purple.

In later years, my friend Joanna, the vicar's wife, agreed that having all these people in the house was more trouble than it was worth. Things came to a head for her when a carer let Edmund escape and he started running down the middle of the road. Despite being instructed by Joanna, the carer had refused to restrain Edmund as it was 'against protocol'.

Our family's breaking point arrived when a carer put James on an ordinary chair without any support, and then left him. He slowly toppled over like a melting ice cream, and would have fallen head first onto the floor if my cleaner, who knew him rather well, hadn't caught him.

None of this helped Tom very much, who simply had to cope with yet more strangers in his house, taking up my time.

The assessments by the staff at the child development centre were finally complete. They reported that James had a mental age of nine months, although he was nearly two. This could no longer be accounted for by the months he had spent in hospital. He couldn't sit up without support, use his left hand or walk, and he was not talking.

The visiting teacher was a wise and experienced woman. She sat me down and said we should be thinking of special schools. 'Does that sound scary?' she asked. I nodded, the tears pricking my eyes. Dr B had mentioned special school but I had shut out the idea. Now it was being put firmly in front of me as a reality. To think of James at a special school gave an indication of the future which I didn't want to consider. Gradually though, she persuaded me that there was a really good special school with a nursery where James could go from two and a half years old. Suddenly an image of empty blue sky sprang into my head.

If James went to a specialist nursery, the responsibility for him learning to walk, talk, keep his glasses on, play, move and eat – responsibilities which had become unbearable –

wouldn't all fall on me. I might have some time for Tom! The visiting teacher said that I should go and see the school, and if I liked it, the next stage would be to get James assessed by an educational psychologist.

The special school was in a suburb of Birmingham which I hadn't been to before. It was well outside the area where James would normally have gone, but special schools had a much broader catchment area than normal schools and children were bussed into this one from all over the city.

I had never been to a special school before and had no idea what to expect. I drove into the entrance in a state of high tension. The site had three schools, one for blind, one for deaf and one for physically disabled children.

As I crossed the threshold there was a battered sign saying 'Blind and deaf children – dead slow'. The physically disabled children weren't referred to in the sign – perhaps because they were mostly in wheelchairs, being pushed by responsible adults and were not a traffic risk.

There was something about the use of the word 'dead' in conjunction with 'blind' and 'deaf' that seemed to encompass the tragedy of the situation. It created a web of rubber bands in my throat which I had not felt since I was travelling in the ambulance to City Hospital, before James was born.

As I went through the big sliding doors at the front, children in a variety of wheelchairs and mobility aids whizzed or staggered by. Signs on the walls showed pictures of speeding wheelchairs with a red cross through them and an exhortation to 'Keep to the left!' This gave me a small inward smile, enough to keep the tears at bay. I later learned that most parents broke down on seeing the school for the first time, and a standard part of the head teacher's job was to administer tea and tissues.

There was equipment everywhere: rooms full of standing frames, therapy benches, specially adapted desks and corridors wide enough to drive a car through, so that the wheelchairs could pass easily. Everything was ramped or on the level. There was also a fully staffed nurses' office, equipped with stretchers, drips, and anti-fitting medication. The head explained to me that all of the children there had some form of physical disability, although it was not always apparent. Some were epileptic, some had cystic fibrosis and others were severely diabetic and needed to be near medical facilities all the time. One child had to attend lessons on a stretcher, followed about by oxygen tanks. Some had bodies which were so different from what I was used to seeing, that even with my experience I found them shocking.

The nursery was full of children like James, some more obviously disabled, some drooling, others whose eyes were not fixed. As a group, even to a sympathetic onlooker such as me, they represented all that as a child myself I would have feared. I realised that while to me James was just my child – beautiful and funny – to everyone else he was one of the most damaged people in society.

It was obvious that this school was where James should go, and so an appointment was booked for an educational psychologist to come and see us after the summer holiday.

*

Our fear of going abroad was still strong after Cyprus, so my mother decided to take us all to a house on the south coast of England for a week.

She had been released from her own burden as a carer when my grandmother, whom she had been nursing, had died. My mother was becoming the rock to which our family could cling, as we floundered about in the open seas of our new-found disabled world.

We set off in our people carrier – it was the first time we had gone any distance with James for over a year.

I noticed that he hated stopping at red lights and would become agitated. He seemed to be soothed when the car began accelerating, and exhilarated when we were going fast. When we got to the holiday house, James seemed desperate to get inside. It was only when we sat him in his special chair in front of his favourite video (*Teletubbies*) that he calmed down. On subsequent days we noticed that the only time he seemed calm was when he was in front of this video. If we tried to go out anywhere, even to the beach, he seemed distressed. I was too tired and busy to consider this behaviour; I had reached the stage where I just dealt with each day as it came and tried to get through it. I was hanging on for James to start nursery and the prospect of a few hours without him.

Eventually the autumn term arrived and the educational psychologist came. He looked just how I imagined a psychologist would look, with a genial face and a slightly crumpled jacket. I took advantage of having an expert on the premises and began by telling him how worried I was about Tom. He suggested a concept called 'special time'. For 20 minutes each day, Tom could have me all to himself, at a time to be agreed in advance between us. During that time, I would be totally available for him and would, with no interruption, play whatever he wanted. It wasn't so easy to execute as I had to abandon James's crammed therapy schedule and try to arrange for someone else to look after him. However, I tried my damndest and when I succeeded it worked very well. I noticed that Tom began to initiate 'special time'. I bit my lip when he wanted yet another 20 minutes of playing trains.

After adding a considerable amount of unexpected value to our lives, the psychologist sat in our living room with a long list of questions on a piece of paper. My impression of his geniality disappeared when he went through the list at breathtaking pace, leaving me far behind. The questions were about what James could and couldn't do, and were painful to contemplate. I became cross and stressed, and when the psychologist left I had a thumping headache.

I didn't realise at the time that he was going through a process, which was simply a means to an end. He was going to show that James was so far behind in his learning that he needed a statement of special educational needs, a piece of paper which would get him into the special school. The piece of paper would take several months to process, so in the meantime I would have to bear my unbearable burden through the winter.

Around that time there was a case in the news about a mother who committed suicide, taking her disabled child with her. It struck me as unbearably sad. Helen Rogan was an occupational therapist who had leapt off a viaduct in Durham with her autistic son, after slashing their wrists with a razor blade. It plucked a strong emotional chord, because she too was in the disabled world and had been struggling. [4]

At that time James had only been diagnosed with cerebral palsy. I remember thinking that I was glad I had a child with just physical disabilities and not autism. How awful, poor woman! What a shame she didn't have more support! I had no idea then that James was also autistic and that within a few years I too would contemplate leaving this world in order to escape the burden created by loving him.

Despite my efforts to look after Tom through 'special time', he was on a timer, which was about to explode, and did so at Christmas.

I had collected him from school a few days before the end of term. He was always grumpy at that time, but I had put this down to the transition period between lessons and home, when there was a change of emotional gear. This time, he sat silent until we got home.

Then he got out of the car, took out his car seat and threw it over the hedge into the road. As he did so, he roared with rage. It was a roar from his guts and soul, and ice water filled my veins as I heard it. He was only four years

4 Nigel Bunyan, The Telegraph online, 5 October 2002.

old. I knew something was very wrong and that something drastic had to be done about it.

We resolved to move Tom to a new school after Christmas, which was much more informal and 'cuddly' than the one he was at. We hoped that with better pastoral support it might help him to deal with the stress he was under at home. We also mentioned our worry about him to Dr A, who referred him to a clinical psychologist. Her letter to the psychologist said:

'Tom's mother is solicitor [sic] but has not worked since she had James and had [sic] put a tremendous amount of work into him. Perhaps not surprisingly the older sibling... is now beginning to show signs of behavioural difficulties which mother probably quite rightly attributes to the fact that he has been pushed out by James in terms of her attention. I think at first he probably just felt this was how life was, but now he is a little older it is becoming different.... Parents are disturbed about Tom's distress and would like some help for him.'

Despite this letter, and chasing by Dr A, the waiting list was so long that it was nearly nine months before we finally got an appointment for Tom to be seen.

In December James had his now customary bout of bronchiolitis and I resigned myself to yet more nights on a camp bed, washing in the sinks of hospital toilets in the morning.

*

In 2001, James had a total of 15 appointments, including those at the child development centre.

Chapter 5
THE INVISIBLE PATH
2002

Although James was now growing up and appeared more robust, we had no opportunity to become complacent about his health. After his admission to hospital for bronchiolitis at Christmas, he could not seem to recover. He had six weeks of continuous ear infections which rendered him feverish, sleepless and skeletal.

I had never seen him so ill since he was born. He wouldn't eat or drink. I had to force water into his body by putting a beaker with a spout into his mouth and gently holding his nostrils. However cruel I felt I was being, I knew that if I didn't do this, James would end up back in hospital, which would cause him even more distress. He seemed to know this and once the spout was in his mouth he would start drinking frantically. When he woke in the night I wouldn't just give him milk, but would sit him in his high chair and spoon fromage frais into his mouth, as it was the only food he would tolerate.

While he was refusing to eat, it was as if my life was on hold. I couldn't think or act while I had an ill and vulnerable child who was starving. All of my energy was spent on getting food and drink into him. Taking James downstairs at 2am, putting the kitchen lights on and sitting there spooning apricot Petit Filous into him ensured that my sleep was completely broken. Gradually my efforts paid off though, and James's weight began to creep up from the bottom centile on the height/weight chart. At one point the nurses had thought he would fall off it altogether.

We had a few weeks of hiatus from worry, and then James

suffered his first seizure since leaving the neonatal unit.

I went into his room one morning and the minute I saw him, even from several feet away, I knew something was very wrong. He was lying almost motionless, making gulping movements with his lips. His eyes were open but unseeing and he was limp and blue-tinged. I was convinced he was dying and dialled 999.

I didn't scream, I had seen so much medical drama at first hand that I was inured to panic, although I had a familiar sensation of ice water in my veins.

An ambulance came, and even the paramedics were upset by what they saw. One of them asked the other if he was OK, as we travelled in the ambulance to City Hospital.

We were admitted into the now very familiar A&E and put back on the children's ward. James came round after a while, and I nearly fainted with relief when I saw that his eyes could once again see and that he recognised me. He reached his hand out and played with my hair. I came to know that when he had these seizures he really needed to feel me, as he couldn't see me and my touch centred him.

A friend who had epilepsy told me that when she had a seizure, the whole world was fragmented and spinning and it was very frightening. From then on whenever I knew James was seizing, I held him and talked to him.

James wasn't diagnosed with epilepsy at this stage. Dr A told me that he was 'allowed two seizures' before they would investigate. Seizures could be caused by a sudden rise in body temperature as well as epilepsy – this was known as a febrile convulsion. An X-ray of James's lungs by Dr B revealed that James had pneumonia. He had a raised temperature on admission, so the seizure was officially recorded as febrile.

I was so anxious to avoid the label of epilepsy that I was relieved that James was ill. The fit could be explained away as a one off, because he was poorly and had a raised temperature. (Oh, the machinations of denial!) A few more nights on a camp bed followed.

*

The physiotherapist had originally diagnosed James as hemiplegic, which meant that he had a weakness down the left side of his body. She had said most hemiplegic children were able to walk in some fashion. This year, however, she decided that the spasticity in James's body didn't just extend down the left side. She thought his right leg and possibly right arm were affected by the cerebral palsy too. He was quadriplegic.

My poor James. We had been assuming that he would be able to move around independently. Now that he was no longer hemiplegic, I didn't want even to think about what this might mean. I didn't dare ask for a new prognosis. I couldn't accept the idea that James might always be in a wheelchair. So I shut the thought in a box, put it in a cupboard and locked the door. I still had hope at that time that he would eventually walk, since he could take steps, as long as one of us held him from behind, to help him balance.

The invisible path, known to the professionals but not to us, flowed on. As James was growing up he needed an orthopaedic consultant, who would keep an eye on the development of his bones and muscles. Because James's brain was constantly causing his muscles to contract, eventually they could deform his growing skeleton.

James's appointment was at a rambling hospital which had started off as an old house. It now had modern wings which had been added on unsympathetically, as well as acres of Portakabins. The cerebral palsy clinic was most unhelpfully tucked away on the first floor, and was only accessible by lots of doubling back through a maze of corridors. The waiting room was tiny and not all the patients could fit into it, since they were all in wheelchairs with carers. A lot of the children were much older than James and some looked unkempt. One girl in particular had long greasy hair. I later found out that at that time, specially adapted facilities at home for disabled children were means tested. If the family didn't qualify for help and couldn't afford it, they would be struggling to keep her clean.

The consultant said that he was satisfied with James's condition, but that he would like to put him on a waiting list for Botox. I was rather taken aback by this, as I had only heard of Botox in connection with face-lifts. He explained that since Botox paralyses the muscles, it could be used to counteract the effects of spasticity. An injection would be made deep into the muscle of James's legs, which could then be stretched more easily. He was a man of few words and rather daunting to deal with. But a friend told me how skilled he was: he was the only surgeon in the area doing this procedure and his patient list went around the world and back.

James had now been issued with some of the little blue shoes which Dr A had mentioned in the neonatal unit, and which had reduced me to tears. They were rather fetching – a bit like baby Dr. Martens. He could crawl around on his own, although we had to roll up his left sleeve, because he dragged his left arm along behind him, and the sleeve would get caught under his body, stopping him in his tracks. He couldn't crawl backwards, so he would find himself in a corner and be unable to reverse. Then he would start calling for me in his own language: 'Gagaga. Gaga gaga ga.'

He had some peculiar eating habits. He didn't like warm food and seemed to prefer sandwiches and crisps to anything else. He wouldn't use a spoon, so he ate everything with his hands. He would have been perfectly capable of using a spoon, as his right hand functioned very well despite the quadriplegia, but he just refused to do so. James had a strong personality and the absence of language didn't stop him from making his views clear. He didn't like having different sorts of food together on the same plate, and would always separate his sandwiches, take out the ham or cheese and put it into a separate pile. To begin with, he would throw anything he didn't want to eat first, onto the floor. Then he would look for it later and have a tantrum when we didn't give it back, flailing his arms and grabbing us if we got within reach. My mother thought he was badly behaved and I should set stricter boundaries. It was hard though, as I had spent so many years trying to get food into his little body that I couldn't bring myself to deny it to him.

Gradually I realised that if I gave James one type of food at a time, he would eat it all. His mealtimes started to resemble a six-course menu in a French restaurant, with tiny plates of different food being served in succession. In the meantime I was trying to maintain a normal meal pattern for Tom, who became used to being denied crisps and given fish fingers and broccoli instead of sandwiches.

I had become friends with Fiona, one of the people I had met through our sessions at conductive education. She told me about a show of equipment for disabled people at the National Exhibition Centre in Birmingham. James was about to get his first Blue Badge so that I could park in disabled parking spaces with him. I was trying to be very brave about this and to demonstrate to myself that I had come to terms with it. So off I went.

The Naidex exhibition was like any other trade event, in that it had glossy brochures, shiny stands and whizzy gadgets to try. There the similarity ended. There can have been no other exhibition like it. For a start, at least half of the visitors were in wheelchairs, leading to a number of traffic jams in the aisles. Then any form of disability which I had not yet heard of was brought vividly to life, as I wheeled James around in his pushchair, happily chomping chocolate buttons.

There were vibrating mats to sit on, to boost circulation. There were cushioned baths that rotated and rolled like fairground rides, jetting water over you. There was a toilet which washed and dried your bottom. There was a device which pushed food into your mouth using a foot operated switch. More sinister, there were reinforced padded tents to calm people with behavioural difficulties and adult-sized cots to stop them wandering around at night. The full range of disabilities was catered for here, filling any gaps in the wildest of imaginations. I remember looking at the padded tents and thinking: 'How awful to have a child that needs that. Thank goodness James isn't like that. That would be much worse than what we have to deal with.' I didn't imagine that in a few years time I would seriously consider buying one of those padded tents.

Although I walked past the tents, I was drawn to a display of bathing equipment designed to make washing easier. Our physiotherapist had ordered James a special bath chair, rather like a plastic car seat with a Velcro seat belt. It helped him to sit up in the water and stay safe, but I still had to lift him in and out of the bath, and my back was beginning to grumble. I went up to a display of baths that could rise up to waist height so you didn't have to bend to wash the patient, and I asked how much it was. When I was told that the basic model without the Jacuzzi was £10,000, I decided I would make do.

At home, I took a child's plastic chair and put it in the shower. The shower head was fixed to the wall very high up so I had to find a way of lowering the stream of water. I bought a plastic funnel and a short length of hosepipe. I jammed the funnel into one end of the hosepipe and using garden twine, I suspended it under the shower head. When the shower was turned on, a manageable stream of warm water came out of the other end of the pipe. Now I could walk James into the shower, holding him under his arms, and I didn't have to lift him over the edge of the bath.

He could sit on the chair with his legs down instead of straight ahead of him, which was much better for his stiff torso. He didn't have to be rained on from a great height; I could gently trail the hose over him, keeping it away from his face.

I felt a mild flush of pride at my inventiveness, but that was to be trumped the second time I gave James his hosepipe shower. In order to wash his bottom I needed him to stand up. I was chatting away to him and said 'Now James, I will have to stand you up so I can wash your bum.' What happened next made the hairs on my neck stand up. It was my first goose bump moment and I vividly recall the feeling ten years later. James grabbed the rail across the door of the shower, and pulled himself to standing. He had understood what I said to him!

Until then I had just talked to him unconditionally, as if he were in a state of prolonged babyhood. I had not had the babble, turning into words, of a non-disabled baby – the babble which led to even the most basic of conversations.

I had known that James could hear me and respond to me, but I didn't know up until then that he understood the meaning of my words. I was choked with emotion and a huge sense of awe at the complexity of him. From then on I talked to James in a different way, looking for any response from him to what I was saying that showed he understood and was answering me.

*

So far, James had escaped the label of epilepsy. However, given his brain haemorrhage, Dr A decided that it would be a good idea to do an EEG anyway. This would detect any abnormal brain waves which showed a tendency to fits. We received an appointment in yet another part of City Hospital. I felt as if I would soon be qualified to give a guided tour of the place.

I had been tasked with getting James there in a state of tiredness so that he would fall asleep while the test was carried out. I thought this would be pretty tricky. How on earth would I get a toddler (who didn't toddle) to sleep, to order? His appointment was at 11am, at least an hour before his usual nap. In the end I woke him an hour earlier in the morning and gave him hardly any breakfast, so that he was starving. Then I took him to hospital with an hour to spare, so he could get used to where he was and the smell of the corridors. It also gave the nurse time to glue coloured electrodes to his head, making him look like an alien hedgehog.

Finally I filled him with cheese sandwiches, before putting a dark blanket over his pushchair and walking him up and down the corridor. It worked, and gave me plenty of time to study another part of the disabled world, which I was hoping heartily then that we would be able to avoid. This was the world of epileptic people.

As I pushed James slowly up and down, I read the leaflets on the corridor walls put up by the Epilepsy Society. There were umpteen varieties of the condition, with strange names. There was petit mal and grand mal; seizures could be atonic and myoclonic; there were secondary generalised seizures and complex partial ones.

Most of the posters were relevant to adults but it still gave me an insight into a condition and a life I had never thought of before. Some people with epilepsy could lose consciousness at any moment – with little or no warning. Some remained conscious but lost control of their bodies completely. Going swimming or climbing, cycling or driving could be life threatening for them.

I felt a tight sensation in my head, a rubber band pulling and tweaking. It was my emotions, being taken to places they didn't want to go. I didn't want to think of a future for James as an epileptic person. I didn't want to think of his future at all at that moment; it was just too painful.

A lady in a white coat saved me. She opened the door and ushered me in, with my sleeping hedgehog. It was surreal, watching the needle on the chart move up and down slowly and gently, recording the activity going on in James's brain. The nurse ended up with a long piece of graph paper with undulations on, similar to those you see in films about earthquakes. She was very firm, though, that someone else would have to look at those undulations before they could come to a decision about James. I tried to get her talking to find out something, but she wasn't letting on. Perhaps she really had no idea. She was very nice though, and we ended up talking about all the therapies I did with James.

'The trouble is,' I said, 'you never know if it makes a difference. I have no way of telling whether he would be just the same if I hadn't done anything at all.' James woke up at this point, and I chatted to him while the nurse removed the coloured electrodes. Then she said to me, 'It does make a difference. You talk to your son. We can always tell. There are children who come in here who just lie there vacantly. No one has ever done anything with them.'

I stored such comments like golden nuggets in a treasure chest deep inside me, to take out and look at when the need arose.

*

The genial psychologist had done his job, and the document called a statement of special educational needs that was the end of the assessment process, was now well under way. The special school decided that James could even start going there without the piece of paper, since it was effectively 'in the post'. This meant that when the statement did arrive, I simply filed it without even reading it. I had no idea how important it would become a few years later.

Thank goodness the visiting teacher had steered me to the school so early. I discovered that the therapy and hospital appointments I had been taking James to were now all held there. I no longer needed to take James to different hospitals and wait in different clinics while he got more and more agitated. I still tried to go to all of James's appointments, but I could leave him in class if the medics overran, rather than trying to entertain him in a waiting room for long periods of time. Doing that was tortuous due to James's very short attention span. Any toys I gave him were simply thrown on the floor and he wasn't interested in books. I usually had to resort to feeding him a long sequence of food to keep him busy.

The school had physiotherapists and speech and language therapists. I had little idea what a speech therapist did, as my exposure to the one at the child development centre had been brief. I assumed that their job was to teach people to speak. It took a while to absorb that speaking and communication were not the same thing. In fact speech and language therapists should really have been called communication therapists. The focus would be on teaching James to communicate rather than articulate, and to use cards and symbols to ask for what he wanted.

Some of the children had talkers, mini computers which could be programmed so that at the touch of a button they would say 'Good morning my name is Jasmine' or 'How are you today?' Even children who could only make tiny movements could operate talkers; there was one girl who used her chin. The staff liked to use Stephen Hawking as an example and point out what his talker had done for him. They regarded their mission as to unlock the person inside the disabled body, to let them out of prison.

The school didn't have an occupational therapist. There had been one attached to the child development centre, whom we had seen briefly. She had obtained some specialist eating equipment for James. He had a mat to go under his plate at mealtimes which was so non slip that you could hardly drag your fingers over it, and it held James's plate like a rock while he ate. He also had some spoons with extra thick handles to make them easier to hold, which curved in towards his mouth rather than being straight.

Other than this, I didn't know what an occupational therapist did. I had vague ideas about someone in an old people's home who held macramé lessons. I later found out that if you can't move, then someone must help you to occupy yourself otherwise you are in a state of torture. You also need someone to consider how you sleep and sit – as there are aids that will make you more comfortable – and whether there are any gadgets which will make you more independent, such as a lift in your home.

Once James was settled into the school, more services came into play. He was getting too big for even the largest disposable nappies I could get from the supermarket and I discovered the world of adult incontinence. This was the place where you cross the line from the normal world of babies, all of whom begin incontinent, to the disabled world, where some remain that way all their lives. James wouldn't always be incontinent of course, I told myself.

The nurses based at the school were in charge of ordering what were now called pads rather than nappies. James was allowed three pads per 24 hours. Luckily for us he didn't drink much, so we managed.

There was also the orthotist. This was the person who helped straighten crooked limbs. He was in charge of providing the little blue shoes and splints. Splints were what used to be called callipers. When I was a child they were made of metal. Now they were plastic, which was cast individually for each child, to be strapped to their lower legs to keep them straight.

At first, when James started at school I would send him in with packed lunches. I was worried that he wouldn't eat school dinners, since he wouldn't touch warm food at home.

The staff drooled over the contents of his lunch box, as I tried ever more inventive ways of getting cold nutrition into him, with cheese sticks, grapes, cashew nuts and dried apricots. There was only one other child who had a packed lunch and I used to drool over *his* food as it included samosas and bajis, which smelt mouth-wateringly good.

As James became used to sitting with the other children

at lunchtime, the staff reported to me that he was looking at what they were eating. They thought they could get him to try cooked food and asked my permission. Within a couple of weeks he was eating stews, mashed potato and even crumbles with custard. Before long he was using a spoon. He wouldn't touch a spoon or warm food at home, but at least the tension I had felt about the effect of his limited diet began to subside, as he was now eating a varied diet at school.

To my great delight, the staff in the nursery fell in love with James after they got to know him. They were intrigued by him and said they had not had another child like him. They told me how on one occasion he had disappeared. They were not sure how he had escaped from the nursery, but they had found him in the toilets, playing with the special large-handled taps and chuckling away as he knelt up at the sink and splashed himself with water. Very early on, though, they discovered that although he formed strong bonds with the adults, he was a danger to other children and would pinch or bite them without hesitation if they were in his way.

After a few weeks when James had been at the school, I realised that I was enjoying a period of calm. His health was stable, the assessment process was over and I now had some sweet time to myself. It didn't take very long for an emotion which I had been too busy to notice, to make itself felt: I was broody again.

I tried to dismiss this feeling. It was simply unthinkable even to contemplate putting ourselves through the ordeal of another pregnancy, now that we knew all too graphically what could go wrong. What would happen to us if we had another disabled child? Even if I had an overwhelming wish for another baby, it wouldn't be fair to Andrew even to raise the subject.

*

In 2002 I filled in a form for disability living allowance for James for the first time. I thought how lucky he was that we lived in a country where the state provided extra money to help him to get around. We planned to get an adapted vehicle that could take his wheelchair. But when the form thudded onto the mat, I found it was 40 pages long. I was used to paperwork and forms, but it took me two days to fill in and it was an emotionally wrenching process.

I had to think in minute detail about how James was different to normal children and to quantify that difference in black and white and time estimates. The form was designed to find out how disabled he was, and it was up to me to spell it out. If I had not realised before then, I realised after I had filled in that form.

'Tell us about the difficulties they have with walking... Has the child's development of social skills been delayed?...

Does the child have difficulties washing, or having a bath or shower?... Does the child need help understanding other people?...

'How many times a day do they need help to make themselves understood by other people?...

'Tell us roughly how long does it take each time? We know this might be difficult but please try to tell us in minutes'. [5]

I finally fell back exhausted and sent the form off.

*

In the summer we once again took our holiday in England, this time choosing Aldeburgh in Suffolk. It was a reasonable holiday, but as with the previous year, James was uncomfortable going anywhere outside the house. I had booked a holiday cottage which I could have sworn it said in the particulars had a video player.

When we arrived, I was dismayed to find no video player.

[5] *Disability Living Allowance Claim Form DLA1A, Department for Work and Pensions, December 2005.*

I checked the brochure and found I had made a mistake. Andrew shrugged and said we would manage. However, we had become so used to James watching videos at home, that we had forgotten how difficult it was to entertain him without them. He was so unable to occupy himself that providing him with a video was the only way the rest of us could have any time to do even the simplest of tasks, such as cook and clean, never mind read or relax.

Although James was only three, the absence of entertainment for him had such an impact on us that I contemplated spending an entire day of our holiday driving to Ipswich and back just to buy a video recorder. Andrew was not in favour, so in the end we took it in turns to have snatches of time 'off duty', wandering round the shops just for an hour or so alone with our own thoughts.

I became anxious again during that holiday about Tom, as his behaviour degenerated quite markedly over a matter of days. He was uncharacteristically naughty and defiant, playing practical jokes such as putting a dead moth into Andrew's cup of tea. My anxiety evaporated however, when I discovered that he was watching *Dennis the Menace* on TV each morning, before Andrew and I got up. When we confronted him he grinned and said he thought it was a great programme!

Despite the absence of a video, there was enough time to relax for the broody emotion to surface again. My resolve not to acknowledge it began to falter and I persuaded myself that we could just take the first step of getting some medical advice to try to assess the risk. After all, that wasn't the same as actually deciding to get pregnant, was it?

My concern for Andrew still held me back. I managed to be strong for most of the holiday but on the penultimate evening there was me, there was Andrew, and there was a bottle of wine. After two glasses the subject slipped out. I was immediately full of regret and trepidation. I told him I would completely understand if he said no to another baby. I wouldn't argue with him, but would accept whatever he said.

To my astonishment, he was all in favour. I was terrified then, as I had anticipated that he would be the brake. I had rehearsed in my mind the scene where he would veto it. I had imagined that I would breathe a sigh of relief and close that door forever. Now we were planning to leap, Thelma and Louise style, into the unknown. After my terror subsided, I was in awe of Andrew's courage. I was made reckless by hormones, he wasn't.

Over the next few days, I realised we shared a deep faith in life, which had somehow been reaffirmed by our decision. Our joy at James's survival had triumphed over the pain of his disability.

We agreed to go and see Miss D, the consultant who had delivered James, as a precaution, to see if another pregnancy was a good idea. She was excited about our plans, which I hadn't expected. She told us that James's early birth was probably due to an infection as there were some signs of this. Another possible cause was 'incompetent cervix' – where the cervix opened prematurely – but this was unlikely since Tom hadn't been born early. In her view, there was no reason we shouldn't try for another baby. She would take extra special care of me during the pregnancy. We left her office elated.

*

By September I was three months pregnant. I was finding carrying James around, particularly upstairs, very tiring and I was worried about my back. I thought of all the equipment I had seen at the Naidex exhibition. I wasn't quite sure who to ask for help. The physiotherapist from the child development centre who had got James his bath seat and high chair was no longer visiting James at home, as he was under the care of the physiotherapists at school. Although they visited our home occasionally, they weren't really involved with his home life. Perhaps an occupational therapist would have been able to help, but there were no occupational therapists at school. The head teacher was very frustrated by this but said it was just impossible to get anyone.

I thought of the occupational therapist from the child development centre who had got James the eating equipment, but then I received a letter telling us that she had left and they would let us know when they had a new person. I was disturbed by this lack of certainty, because I wanted to try to get some new equipment in place before I became too big with my pregnancy.

I rang the hospital and discovered that I could self-refer James to the central occupational therapy service in our area. I did so by phone but didn't get a response for two months, so I rang them again and this time wrote as well. I got a letter back which said they couldn't tell me when I would get any help.

'…Your request for an assessment has now been given careful consideration and your details put on our waiting list.

'This is a service for which there is a very high demand and at present, we are unable to tell you when you are likely to be seen. However, you will be contacted with a definite appointment time in due course and we will do all we can to keep any delay to a minimum.

'The staff are making every effort to deal with everyone fairly and as quickly as possible but they will give the highest priority to people who are terminally ill, who cannot leave hospital or who are in immediate danger.'

I raised the subject with Dr R, another consultant who was seeing James in clinic at his school. She groaned and shook her head. She told me that her patients with Duchenne muscular dystrophy, who she could predict would become unable to walk, could not be put on the waiting list for adaptations until they showed signs of being disabled. Then they might have a two-year wait until they had the equipment they needed.

In November, Dr A referred James to a clinical psychologist. The school was concerned about his aggressive behaviour. He could not be left unattended around other children as he might bite them. Dr A also thought James's approach to food, which was very rigid at home, could have a psychological cause. Tom had still not been seen, so I now had two children waiting to see a psychologist.

Despite the fact that James ate cooked food at school, his eating at home was still very limited. I became concerned again about his diet and the school nutritionist agreed to order a blood test. It was an awful experience, because James had developed a phobia for hospitals (who could blame him) and was very unhappy at being dragged to one first thing in the morning with no breakfast (he had to be nil by mouth). He had skinny, bony arms and the phlebotomist, a clinician trained in taking blood, struggled to find a vein. James struggled back and I had to restrain him while he tried to arch his back and cried. The result came back normal though, and I felt physically lighter in the knowledge that he really was getting enough nutrition.

By New Year's Eve I was 25 weeks pregnant. All had gone very well with the pregnancy and I was feeling smug and confident. I was carrying a girl – the cherry on the cake after two boys. I was rushing around preparing for some friends who were coming for supper when I suddenly remembered that I was due to go into City Hospital late afternoon for a routine scan. Damn! I picked up the phone to rearrange it. I was sure another week wouldn't make any difference. Then I put the phone down again. I shouldn't really take any chances, and it wouldn't take too long. I should be back home by 6pm.

An hour later I was lying on my back with cold jelly on my abdomen, straining to see the grey blobby images of my daughter on the monitor. There was a quiet but distinct gasp from the ultrasonographer. 'What is it?' I asked. 'Nothing', she replied, 'I just need to make a phone call.' Five minutes later she came in carrying a telephone with Miss D on the end of it. 'Jane, you must stay flat on your back,' said Miss D. 'Flat on your back and don't move.'

*

In 2002 James had nine hospital appointments and four emergency admissions.

Chapter 6
DÉJÀ VU

2003

Far from being home by 6pm, I remained in hospital for two months, hardly daring to breathe. My cervix had opened prematurely and the balloon in which my daughter was safely stored was threatening to burst - something we now knew must have happened with James. The danger had only been picked up this time because Miss D had ordered extra-detailed scans for me.

At first I was on a ward, but within a few hours I was put in a single room with its own bathroom. I was on bed rest and I didn't leave that room for eight weeks. The staff from the neonatal unit visited me and assured me they were all on stand-by for my little girl. They would keep a cot for her and wouldn't let her go to Edinburgh, as might have been the case with James.

Through the mists of deep shock that I was experiencing for a second time, I turned again to the Being that I had begged to save James's life and with whom I had kept in touch since then. This time I felt I had a bit more bargaining power. 'I promise to pray,' I said to God, 'as long as she isn't born today.'

I began to read the Bible, which I hadn't really done before. I hadn't realised that it was a collection of books. I had always started with page one of the Old Testament, which seemed to involve a lot of people begetting and begatting, and after a few pages of this I had given up. Now in the hospital, I started with the New Testament and read the Gospels. I realised they were four eyewitness accounts of Jesus' life on Earth. Four witness statements! As a lawyer that appealed to me. The hairs on my neck rose with the similarity of those accounts, and yet the fact they had obviously been written by different people.

I decided I was going to pray for a miracle. The praying was helpful in dealing with the terror I was feeling.

I only allowed myself to get up once each day, to have a shower. I looked forward to that shower so very much. After the stultifying warmth of the mattress and the sheets, the sensation of running water and the tang of citrus shower gel kept me sane.

The only other sensory pleasure I had was eating. Miss D had told me that we needed to try to get the baby as big as possible before she was born, which was likely to be soon, so I started to eat and eat.

Kind friends were worried I would be bored; they couldn't imagine being trapped in bed all day with nothing to do. How could I explain to them that it's difficult to be bored when you are in a state of absolute fright? 'You could do a language course' said one. 'I'll bring you some cross-stitch' offered another. I had no idea what cross-stitch was, but she returned with a little kit, a sort of sewing by numbers, which if followed correctly would result in a bookmark with a vase of roses stitched on it. It was another good way of keeping away the terror, although I was no seamstress. My wonky roses looked more like Triffids.

We decided to call our daughter Elizabeth. After a few days had gone by, she was showing no signs of impatience and daily scans indicated she was getting nice and fat, as was I. The staff were surprised and pleased and my terror began to lessen a little. Friends who had sent shocked cards and letters were beginning to feel they could visit and I was beginning to feel that I was up to seeing them. Wonderful women sat in my room and brought me nuts, chocolate and sandwiches, and I ate and ate. One friend was a news reporter and she rushed in one evening after work, looking

89

very glamorous in a black suit. When she had gone I had a deputation of nurses, saying 'Was that really Sandy Barton?!' Until then, I had simply seen Sandy as a friend. I was amused to find that a little stardust had rubbed off on me. I became a celebrity by association.

I still wouldn't get out of bed unless I absolutely had to, and I still prayed a lot. Now I was emboldened and began to tag extra requests onto my prayers, not just 'Please don't let Elizabeth be born early' but 'Please give her a happy life'. After a while I became outrageous and added on 'Please make her beautiful and clever, with a lovely voice', a bit like the fairies in *Sleeping Beauty* who had three gifts to bestow. In my flippancy, I was simply struggling not to surrender to the blackest of emotions. The horror of my situation and that of my threatened daughter could only be kept at bay by sleeping, eating and praying. When the reality broke through, as it did every now and then, it threatened to destroy me.

One evening a consultant on duty, whom I only met once, sat on my bed for a long chat. He told me that if James's brain damage had been caused by the hospital (which it hadn't) then we would have had hundreds of thousands of pounds for his care for the rest of his life. By contrast, children whose disability was nobody's fault received nothing. My response was instant. 'Money or not, I couldn't have borne it if James's disability were someone's fault' I said, 'It would have been intolerable.'

After a few weeks, when Elizabeth was at 30 weeks gestation, I felt I could move around a little more. I knew that the crucial time was between 24 –28 weeks, when every day made a real difference. Thirty weeks was still far from ideal, but it was another planet from 25. I began to go and get my own food from the trolley at mealtimes, rather than expecting the staff to bring it, and so I solved the mystery of the treacle pudding. Every time I had selected it from the daily menu I had been disappointed by the arrival of a lump of plain sponge and custard. When I saw the catering tin I realised that the pudding had been made upside down, with the syrup on the bottom of the tin, which is where it had stayed.

I also started choosing the Asian food, to the amusement of the women serving it, as spicy bean curry was so much more interesting than shepherd's pie.

It was very hard not seeing James and Tom, except for a short visit at weekends. Andrew came in most nights. He brought in a card which the teachers had helped James to make. I was doing very well at not crying, but when I saw this card, great deep sobs racked my chest and I had to cling to Andrew. The card was covered in photos of James doing activities at school and said:

'Hello Mummy
I thought you might like to know what a nice day I have had at school today. I had a ride on a bike before dinner. Dad made me a lovely lunch today and I ate it all up. This afternoon I had music therapy and then I played in the tent with tunnels.'

Part of its poignancy was that it gave James a voice he didn't usually have. But I knew he missed me; he used to cling to me and cry when Andrew tried to take him home. Andrew was exhausted, trying to do everything I normally did as well as go to work. My mother, who also worked full time, drove up and down the motorway from Surrey every Friday to help him at weekends. Tom was just still and silent.

I couldn't afford to think about what this situation was doing to all of them. I was in some primeval place, where all I could do was to try to protect Elizabeth from the fate that had befallen James.

One day I had a message that someone from the occupational therapy service had called. They were offering to do a telephone questionnaire to see if we were entitled to a grant for adaptations to the house, before they came to assess us formally. I was pleased that we had finally heard from someone, although I hadn't realised that help was means tested. I told the person what they wanted to know and he told me, on an informal basis, that we wouldn't currently qualify for any financial help. He would keep us on the system, though, in case anything changed. We would also be entitled to a visit to give us advice about the equipment we might need for James and where to get it.

A few months later, we got a letter from the occupational therapy service which was identical to the one we had received the previous year. They still were unable to say when they could formally assess us. So even if we had qualified for financial help, they still weren't in a position to begin the process, nearly nine months after I had first self-referred!

When I was 33 weeks pregnant I was allowed home. I had become so institutionalised that I didn't want to leave. I would have been happy to stay there on my bed, watching TV, doing cross-stitch and being fed. However, I was needed at home, so that wasn't an option. I noticed that for the first few hours in the house I was treated like a china doll, but very quickly everyone reverted to type, expecting me to be mother again.

Elizabeth was induced when I was 38 weeks pregnant. Miss D didn't want to take any chances with her and wanted a planned delivery. Her birth wasn't trouble free though. On the day I was admitted for her to be born, the maternity unit at City Hospital had one of its busiest days ever. By 6pm I had been waiting for nine hours. Miss D arrived exhausted and apologetic. I would have to wait until the morning!

I persuaded Miss D to let me go home, and the next day I was rewarded with an almost silent delivery suite. My waters were broken artificially and labour began. I was so scared that I was determined not to be in pain at any point if I could manage it so I opted for an epidural. This was a mistake since it slowed the birth down as it had with James, and Elizabeth got stuck. Miss D had to perform a ventouse delivery and suddenly the room was full of people, just as it had been with James. Only this time Elizabeth lay happily on my stomach, big eyes open and calmly looking around. She took a brief two sucks of breast and then she was handed over to Andrew. He began to sing to her 'Elizabeth you're my teddy bear', and I realised that there were a lot of moist eyes looking on.

Now I had to face up to the bargain I had driven with God in hospital. I had become rash and added the promise of a speech of thanksgiving in church to the daily prayers I had offered for Elizabeth's safe deliverance. Still, who knew what might happen if I didn't keep my bargain. So two months later I waddled up to the lectern (I was still very large), feeling self-conscious. Taking a deep breath, I just managed to get to the end of a pre prepared speech before my throat closed up.

I was now re-immersing myself in the lives of my two older children. Tom seemed a lot calmer at his new school and was relieved to have me back. James had his appointment with the clinical psychologist to discuss his unusual eating patterns and aggressive behaviour.

The clinical psychologist talked about how disabled children often had a greater need for routine because of their vulnerability. She thought James liked getting a reaction to his behaviour, so we should try not to react when he hurt us. She thought he might get bored of it if there was no response and we agreed to give it a try. It takes some self-restraint though, not to gasp when someone pinches you with all their might. It was beyond Tom's ability and he learnt to keep well out of James's reach.

Father's Day arrived and Tom came home with a card he had made at school. James, however, came home with nothing.

I was puzzled by this as when I was in hospital I had

received a Mother's Day card from both children. I asked the staff at James's school why he hadn't made one. The answer came back 'Most of our children don't have fathers around.'

I later found out that marriage breakdown rates are much higher where there is a disabled child. Official statistics are hard to find, but many people I know quote anecdotal evidence of 80 per cent divorce rates among parents of children with special needs. Perhaps not surprisingly, as women are usually the main carers of non-disabled children, it is the mothers who often remain as the main care-givers of disabled children. So the school had decided that it was inappropriate to have a session creating Father's Day cards, when most of the children didn't have dads around to give them to.

*

In the June half term I took all three children to stay with Katherine, my London GP friend. She was very fond of getting the children into the open air, whatever the weather. She had once persuaded me to stay on in a National Trust garden, after it was officially closed due to icy conditions. We slithered along frozen paths and hid from the wardens who were trying to round up the last of the visitors.

On this occasion it was much warmer, and we were wandering the grounds of a stately home. James and Elizabeth were in pushchairs. I was pushing Elizabeth and Katherine was pushing James. He was just about to get his first wheelchair. I was telling Katherine about it as we ambled along the rhododendron walk. I was getting a bit emotional as I told her about a sticker I had bought for the back of the car which said 'wheelchair passenger'. I lost concentration and was brought back to focus by Katherine, who was usually very polite, yelling 'Fucking hell!' In a lapse of concentration I had let go of Elizabeth's pushchair and forgotten to put the brake on. It was rolling at an increasing pace towards a steep drop covered in beech leaves. Fortunately Katherine was very sporty, and she leapt forward like a gazelle to save the day.

I was now dealing with a new baby while James, although nearly four, also couldn't walk or talk. It was like having two babies at once. I bought a special needs double buggy which could take the two of them together. The new one was so wide though that I couldn't fit it through most doorways.

I worked out there were only two places I could go from home and that was to the park or to the shopping centre, which had sliding doors into all the shops.

I couldn't get a rain cover to fit the buggy. The mother I had bought it from told me she used to put her children in bin bags when it rained. She said she didn't care what people thought. I knew what she meant. Daily life could be such a struggle but most people had no idea. If you tried to maintain normal standards just to keep up appearances, you would go under. It didn't really matter what they thought. Or, as a poster on the wall of Tom's school said:

*'Those who matter don't mind
and those who mind don't matter.'*

James's need for supervision was increasing as he got older. He was now using the video player to manipulate the videos, making *Teletubbies* run back and forth endlessly at his will. He was totally engrossed in this, which made entertaining him easier, but we were all too dependent on the tapes working. We briefly flirted with using DVDs, but James liked biting them and then they were useless, so we had gone back to the more robust videos. The video player took such a battering that we had to replace it once a month with a new one, sometimes even more often. The heads would need cleaning and if this wasn't done regularly, the tapes would get contaminated and *Teletubbies* would be grainy and spotty.

Sometimes the tapes broke, and the video player stopped working. James would become hysterical then, and lash out. We began to dread these episodes and took extreme steps to avoid them. We bought a stock of second-hand video players and had one on stand-by in case another one broke. I got used to opening up the innards of the machines to extract broken bits of tape and to try to clean both tape and machine and put it back together. The whole process took up hours of my time.

Just before the summer holidays began, James had another seizure, this time at school. I had become used to seeing him fit and giving him emergency medication. I had adopted a policy of keeping him at home if at all possible now that I had Elizabeth, as the logistics of having to be in hospital overnight were horrendous. This time I had no choice, as the school nurses called an ambulance and he was taken straight to City Hospital. When the head teacher rang to let me know I shrank with dismay.

I contemplated the next few hours in hospital coping with a small baby (Elizabeth) and a six-year-old tired from school (Tom), while I sat by James's bedside until Andrew could come home from work. I could not prevent myself being furious with the head teacher, until she interrupted me and said 'JANE HE WAS TURNING BLUE!'

I realised how blasé I had become about James's condition, and how my circumstances were forcing me to take risks which would otherwise be unthinkable.

Tom finally had his appointment with the clinical psychologist. He had had to wait for nearly nine months. By then the episode where he had thrown the car seat over the hedge after school in a fit of rage, seemed a long time in the past. Although I wished his life were a lot different, I didn't have the gut-twisting feeling about him that I had had before. The clinical psychologist was satisfied that he was doing OK too, so I took a rare moment to appreciate something in our family that was going well.

*

That summer we decided rather nervously to go abroad. We thought we could cope with a trip to northern France with my mother along to help. It was wonderful to taste proper baguettes and croissants again, to sip rosé wine in street cafés. However, drunk with the excitement of leaving England, we were over-ambitious in our plans. We stayed in four different bed and breakfasts and two different holiday cottages, with miles of driving in between. James became unsettled and distressed, sleeping very badly and crawling around the bedroom at night.

We had to give him a room to himself, and put his mattress on the floor so that having shuffled off it he could get back onto it when he was tired. We had to barricade the door so that he couldn't get out. Despite these measures we all had very disturbed sleep from James's noise.

When we got home, we had just reached the familiar suburbs of Birmingham when James began to yelp in a way I had not heard before and to look intently at his surroundings. He was literally crying with joy and I realised then that he couldn't believe he was home again. I once again marvelled at how aware he was and realised that I had underestimated his understanding of his environment. I also felt a pang of guilt that I had put him through an upheaval which he obviously couldn't cope with, and I resolved not to do it again.

The summer dragged on with a ribbon of domestic chores: feeding the children; cleaning up James; washing the dishes and the clothes; not ironing because as long as the clothes were clean I could live with crumpled. One day even the ironing got done, oddly enough by Sandy.

In an act of supreme altruism, she passed on the

opportunity to interview someone famous, in order to keep a date for coffee with me. She stood in my garden ironing my family's clothes, while I sewed and we chatted. My spirits rose to have another adult around who was cheerful and sympathetic. My good friends were golden nuggets and when my mother and Andrew couldn't be there, their warmth kept a little fire going inside me, which would otherwise have gone out.

Just before the autumn term started, the speech and language therapist from James's school came to pay a home visit. I was very pleased to see her because when I had come out of hospital with Elizabeth, I had noticed that James was using his eyes to point to things rather than his hand, which he had done previously. The staff had said that there were a lot of children in class who couldn't move their limbs, so eye pointing had been adopted as the norm.

'But James can move and point with his right hand!' I had said. 'He will always have his hand on the end of his arm. If he can learn to sign then that will be much better than eye pointing.' Looking back, it is obvious to me now that the fact James had adapted to the way the whole class was communicating, and had changed from hand signs to eye pointing, was evidence that this child knew what was going on.

The speech and language therapist agreed with me that eye pointing was not appropriate for James and wanted to trial a technique called picture exchange communication system or PECS. It involved teaching the child to ask for something by handing a picture of it to the carer. What would motivate James most, she wanted to know.

'Crisps' I said. 'Salt and vinegar crisps.' She took all the crisps out of a bag and gave me the empty packet. 'You have to give me the packet' she said. 'I then take it and give you a crisp in return.' We did this twice to show James. 'Now it's James's turn' she said. 'It will probably take him quite a lot of goes to get this. The average is 20 goes, but some children need 100.'

James was looking longingly at the crisps. He reached for one but the therapist wouldn't give it to him, so he picked up the packet and gave it to her. She and I both felt a wave of goose bumps. Then he did it again and again, getting crisps as fast as he could eat them. 'I've never seen a child get it straight away' she gasped.

I could have hugged her. I had an ally. Now someone else knew just how well James understood what we were saying.

*

In September James had his first Botox injections, at a hospital we hadn't been to before. We had to arrive for 7.30am and James was nil by mouth. He kept crawling off his hospital bed and picking up bits of discarded plastic from the floor to chew. In the end the staff brought a large cot with metal bars and we put him in it. He kept pulling himself up to stand, but he didn't have a firm footing on the mattress and wobbled precariously. I was worried he would fall over and crash his head against the bars. I couldn't leave him for a second. He thought it was very funny, and when he wasn't standing, bunny hopped around in the cot, giggling and chewing the rails.

The consultant was prepared to treat him while he was in the cot but first he had to have a sedative. He needed to be still and sleepy when they injected the poison deep into his legs. Other parents, even the nurses, watched in horror as I held his nostrils shut to make him swallow the sedative. I knew that if I didn't do this, he would obediently open his mouth for the spoon, hold the medication on his tongue for a moment then spit it out again as soon as I took the spoon away.

The sedative didn't knock him out as much as I thought it would, it just made him slightly woozy, and so he couldn't crawl properly and looked a bit drunk. I held his legs while a very long needle went in, and a blob of bright red blood welled up when it was withdrawn.

I had seen the other parents looking at James as he chattered in his cot like a monkey and realised how very different he looked from any of them. Although there were a lot of children with physical disabilities or learning difficulties, James stood out as being more damaged than any other. I felt cold and more than sad – I felt unreal. It was the beginning of a deep depression.

The occupational therapy service finally caught up with itself and a therapist turned up at the house to assess it for James's needs. I was pleased to see him as even though we would have to pay for the adaptations, he would be able to give us expert advice about what to get and where to get it.

We had a particularly interesting conversation because he was Kenyan, from the Kamba tribe south of Nairobi, and I had done voluntary work in that part of Kenya in my late teens.

We talked about the vivid red soil, the huge green cacti and the local beer, called (appropriately for Africa) Tusker. He told me about the occupational therapy system in Birmingham that meant any building works were means tested and there was a waiting list of two years. However, he could get anything for me that wasn't fixed to the house, for free.

So, he could order portable hoists but not those attached to the ceiling. We could have portable bath support chairs but not one of the £10,000 up and down baths that I had seen at the Naidex exhibition.

I asked about beds that went up and down. I wanted one for James that we could lower to the floor at night so he could crawl on and off it, but one that I could raise in the day when I was changing him, so that I didn't have to bend. My back was in shreds after carrying James and now a baby around for a combined total of four years. He said that he couldn't get me a bed but I could try my GP. I asked my surgery about this but they weren't able to help. I later found out that several doctors had gone to great lengths to try and find out where I could get a 'hospital' bed, which would cost nearly £1,000, but without success. Still, several bits and pieces ordered by the therapist arrived over the next few weeks, which made life easier.

During the autumn term, I noticed that it was getting harder and harder to get James ready to be picked up by his school bus in the morning. The physical tasks of feeding and washing him could be done to order, what was becoming very stressful was managing the psychology.

The bus collected several children and its arrival time could vary by as much as 20 minutes. It would only wait for five minutes, though, if we were late. Occasionally it was early but often, if there was a problem with the traffic, it was late. James would expect his morning to follow a predictable sequence of events, so if the normal routine was disrupted he would become hysterical, attacking me. He would refuse to get into his wheelchair, which made it impossible to load.

I could have put him in his wheelchair before he even left his bedroom. He would have been captive then. But he was able to move around the house without the chair. He could slide down the stairs on his stomach and crawl into the kitchen. With every sinew, I was determined to keep him as mobile and independent as possible. That meant only using his wheelchair for transporting him outside the home.

In October he had yet another seizure – the fourth of the year. This time something was different. I went to get James up in the morning and discovered him lying in a pool of sick.

He was very blue and moaning quietly. This was not a time to be blasé. I shouted to Andrew to dial 999 and, used to the drill by now, he didn't ask questions. He later told me what it was like going into work and explaining that he was delayed because one of his children had stopped breathing.

He would say how James had gone blue and we had had to call the ambulance. There would be a stunned silence while his colleagues tried to absorb the enormity of this one event, unaware that it was only one of many that had preceded it.

The paramedics came and gave James oxygen, but once he was sedated and pink they were happy to leave. James lay on the sofa for the rest of the morning. He moaned intermittently but, unusually, didn't open his eyes. It took me two hours to work out that he must have acid in them from the vomit. I rinsed them as best I could and gradually little bloodshot peeps came from under his lids.

Used as I was to trauma, this spooked me to the point where I thought we must do something to stop these fits. I had come to a point of acceptance, where even if his condition were called epilepsy, we had to do something about it.

In November, Dr A saw James in clinic and told us that a second EEG had come back inconclusive, so for the time being he would remain a 'non-epileptic person'. However, she was becoming concerned about other aspects of his behaviour. She said in a letter to the GP:

' *As far as his behaviour is concerned, school feels he is developing more unusual behaviours, flicking his hands upwards, rocking, putting his hands down his trousers, putting his fingers up his nose...* '

I had an uneasy feeling. I was so used to James, so immersed in him, that I couldn't see him as others saw him. I was incapable of assessing him independently. I still knew though, that his behaviour was different to what I, or anyone I knew, was used to.

*

In 2003 James had 18 hospital appointments and two emergency admissions.

Chapter 7
MELTDOWN
2004

During the first few months of 2004, aged well over four years old, James had his first serious poo episode. It probably wouldn't have happened if he had been continent, but he wasn't. The incontinence of babies is something of horror to most people who aren't their parents; the incontinence of older children is unspeakable.

I entered the playroom where he watched his videos, and thought the odour of excrement was more pungent than usual, although I was fairly inured to a ripe pad. Poo is pretty disgusting even when contained in a nappy, but this had emigrated far beyond its normal boundaries. As I got nearer to James I saw with disbelief that he had poo all over his right hand and his face and mouth. I realised that he had put his hand into his nappy and had been actually eating his own faeces. It was also all over the video player, the table he was sitting at, the bench he was sitting on, and the TV screen he was licking. He had picked up several videos which were also plastered in brown. A cold dull feeling stopped me in my tracks for a minute, as I stood and looked at this awful scene. There is something so base about excrement. The IRA hunger strikers smeared it on the walls of their cells in the Maze prison in the 1970s. It engenders universal opprobrium. Children who have accidents when they are toilet training quickly pick up on this disgust from their parents. Later the first naughty word they use is usually 'poo'. 'You are a poo poo head! Ha ha!'

More surreal, was that James was oblivious to the unacceptability of what he had done. There was no toddler defiance 'Look what I've done Mummy, so there!' He used his pooey hand to pick up another video and asked me to change the one he was watching, even offering to give me a pooey kiss at the same time.

Dealing with a 'poo fest', as Andrew came to call it, was another matter. Excrement is surprisingly hard to clean up. Once it leaves the body it ceases to be sterile and becomes a serious contaminant. Cleaning it off a bouncing child who wants to keep watching TV is quite a challenge. The whole process of disinfecting James, the equipment and the playroom, would take an hour or so. We had to write off numerous video players where faeces had become stuck in the buttons and couldn't be cleaned out satisfactorily. We once had to throw away an entire carpet where some had been trodden into the pile. We kept a multipack of brightly coloured children's toothbrushes for a disposable clean of James's mouth. After a few poo fests we built up a disinfectant armoury that Porton Down would have been proud of.

We had latex disposable gloves, various coloured brushes for different stages of the process, and industrial-sized air fresheners. Andrew bought a cranberry scented one at Christmas, so unfortunately for me, the smells of cranberries and poo are now forever intertwined ...

Often these episodes happened in the early hours of the morning. James usually woke at 4am and bounced vigorously on his bed. This of course had the same effect that exercise does on us all, and so we would find ourselves confronted with a bedroom poo fest. By the time we had finished cleaning up it was impossible to get back to sleep before we had to get up again. We ended up taking shifts, with me handling the weekdays and Andrew the weekends.

On weekdays I would walk around in the kind of stupor familiar to parents of newborn babies. I would get the children off to school, then spend the morning doing housework in a slow, zombified state, longing for noon to come so that I could go back to bed for a couple of hours before they came home again.

*

In March I had a meeting with the head of James's nursery.

It was one of those beautiful English spring days when, for the first time that year, the sun shines warmly enough to allow you to sit outside.

Perhaps it was the peace of being away from the classroom or the heat on our skin that made the meeting feel more relaxed and expansive than usual. Anyway, we were chatting about James: how he could take your breath away with flashes of intelligence; how loving he was; and how he would attack other people or himself when he was distressed. The head paused for a second, 'I've never had a child quite like him' she said. 'There's something about the way he behaves ...' she hesitated, 'some of the things he does make me wonder if he is autistic.' The minute she said the word 'autistic' an image came into my mind of a slot machine in which all the lemons had just lined up in a row. She had hit the jackpot.

I thought of James's obsession with routine and his endless manipulation of *Teletubbies* back and forth; his dislike of going anywhere he didn't know or doing anything different, except when he knew he was on a school trip. I thought of the way he separated his food into different types. I had friends with autistic children and so was familiar with some of the characteristics. But, preoccupied as I had been with teaching James to walk, talk and eat with a spoon, I had never applied them to him.

The familiar cold dull feeling came over me. I knew somewhere very deep, in the part of me that didn't use words, that the head of the nursery was right. So now I had a child with cerebral palsy, who had seizures and was probably epileptic and also had autism. What had I done to

105

deserve this truly terrible situation? What had James done? I didn't cry. I seemed to have lost the ability to cry.

I went home and starting reading about autism. I found out about the 'triad of impairments' – the three main hallmarks of autistic spectrum disorder – difficulty with social communication, difficulty with social interaction and difficulty with social imagination. James slotted pretty clearly into all of them.

There was only one aspect of his character that didn't fit the box and that was his sense of humour. Autistic people were supposed to have difficulty with humour. James was always laughing and teasing the people looking after him.

Every morning at breakfast time he would point to a cupboard in the kitchen where I kept the crisps and make a noise meaning 'Give me some!' I would say 'No James, you can't have crisps for breakfast!' in mock horror. Then he would giggle. Eventually I moved the crisps into another room and showed him they were no longer in the kitchen, but he would still ask for them every morning just to hear me say 'No!'

His humour made him easy to love, which I was very pleased about, for his sake. Even at that stage I knew he would always need carers other than me, and if they found him easy to love he would have a better life.

I prepared a note for Dr A, setting out how James's behaviour measured up against the triad of impairments. We were due to meet a few days later. She said that on the basis of what I had written she would diagnose James as autistic. She said it was usual for children to be referred for further assessment, but she couldn't see how in James's case that would get him any more help, and it would simply be time-consuming and emotional for me. She would, however, get me another appointment with the clinical psychologist, who could suggest some strategies for dealing with him.

I told the psychologist how when we were in the car and had to stop for a red light, James would go berserk and lash out at Tom and Elizabeth, or hurt himself. I had to tie his hand down to prevent him.

I told her about the fact that he regularly woke at 4am and bounced for a couple of hours before going back to sleep. I told her of the poo fests. I mentioned his distress at doing virtually anything outside the house, which was beginning to make weekends and school holidays impossible. I told her how he would, however, go anywhere on school trips without fuss.

She thought he might be suffering from sensory deprivation because he couldn't move around easily and wasn't able to touch things. She suggested creating a touch panel with different fabrics which could be hung by his bed at night so that he could stroke it.

She suggested that I should also take photos of the places we visited, so that I could explain in advance where we were going. She advised having a fixed routine throughout the holidays, so that at all times of the day James knew what to expect. Finally, she recommended inventing little ditties to sing at traffic lights to keep him calm when we stopped.

I could see that what she was saying was brilliant advice, but a great weariness settled on me as I mentally added all those tasks on to keeping everyone fed and clean, while I remained in a state of chronic sleep deprivation. How could I have a rigid routine throughout weeks and weeks of school holidays, with a baby, a seven-year-old and James to occupy and care for?

I never did make a touch panel and sticking to a rigid holiday routine was impossible, but I took photos of some of the places we went to most often, which seemed to help James a lot. I had to get the photos laminated or he would chew them into a pulp. The ditties also worked. Tom and Elizabeth got used to me singing 'Red means stop and green means go' in a nursery rhyme voice, until they were sick of it. But at least we didn't have to strap James's hand down any more in the car to prevent him lashing out when we stopped.

One social worker I met years later told me of a mother whose autistic son used to pull her hair when they were out in their car and had to stop at red lights. She took to wearing a wig to protect her poor scalp. This was more effective than she had anticipated, because the son was so spooked by the sudden change in his mother's hair that he sat in silent fear and left her alone.

*

As summer approached, I viewed the school holiday with dread. I was wondering what on earth to do, when the child development centre found James a play scheme. It was held in a nursery in a deprived area of Birmingham and that summer he went for several weeks. It gave me an insight into yet another world – the world of social deprivation. The nursery was heavily subsidised and ran all through the holiday, to look after children from households that were struggling. It opened at 7.30am with a breakfast programme, gave the children a cooked lunch at 11.30am, and sent them home at 4pm after a sandwich tea. I was told that for some children the only regular meals they got were those they ate there.

There was a great emphasis on giving the children a social framework. Basic manners and respect for other people were reinforced all the time. It was a wonderful place that practised genuine inclusion, and where no effort was spared to make James part of the class. There was a cuddly girl who looked after him and he adored her. When the scheme had finished I took him back a few weeks later to say hello. As he entered the room and saw her, he blushed noticeably and lowered his eyes. She was so touched by this unexpected sign of closeness that she too blushed bright red. I was almost in tears that my little disabled son was so emotionally aware.

Knowing now of James's anxiety about change, we didn't dare to go abroad that summer, and instead booked a house on the East Coast at Old Hunstanton, only three hours drive away from Birmingham. Even then, instead of looking forward to the holiday I anticipated it with dismay. There would be no respite from James and he would be even more difficult to deal with out of his normal environment. We would be struggling to give the other children anything resembling a normal family break. As for any relaxation for Andrew and me, that was out of the question.

Some neighbours of ours also happened to be in Norfolk at the same time and we made a provisional arrangement to meet up. We set up a time to call when we could both get a mobile signal, but they missed it. When they eventually rang, they were glowing with the pleasure of their day on the beach. 'We've just been for an evening swim' said the wife. 'Sorry we didn't ring earlier but the water was so warm and we were having a lovely time.' Then the signal cut off. They tried to ring us back but Andrew and I were shamefully jealous and ignored them. In one casual phrase they had underlined everything we couldn't achieve in our holiday. It wasn't that we couldn't swim in the sea – it was that the effort it would involve was exhausting just to contemplate. We also had no enjoyment in anything. The usual spikes of pleasure at something even as simple as the smell of cut grass or a good ice cream, just didn't happen now. We went through each day with an unvarying feeling of dreariness.

While we were in Hunstanton, a swarm of hover flies settled over the town for two days. When we ventured out at all we were covered by hundreds of them. It felt like a biblical plague, and couldn't have been more symbolic of the pestilence which we felt was blighting our lives. We were going deeper and deeper into a swirling fog of depression which, before we knew it, would leave us stumbling and unable to see.

During the second week of the holiday, I was buying some sweets in a seaside shop that sold buckets and spades and sticks of rock. A postcard caught my eye. It had a close up picture of a beach hut on it.

There was something so comforting about the beach hut. It was small and private, painted white with a yellow door. It had only a sand dune below, with a bit of Marram grass. Above it was clear blue sky. I imagined going inside the bare, white wooden interior and closing the yellow door. In my beach hut there was no one else and nothing, except a bed for me to lie down on while I listened to the sound of the sea and the gulls overhead.

I bought the picture, framed it and put it on the kitchen wall, next to the sink. When I was overwhelmed with everything I would look at it and transport myself into the hut for a few moments.

*

That autumn I had what used to be called a nervous breakdown. I knew something was very wrong when I was sitting on a bus and tears started to pour down my face. I couldn't stop them at all. I didn't know why I was crying – only that everything felt terrible and terrifying, as if life were a black tidal wave, rearing up at me.

The next day, while Tom and James were at school, I took Elizabeth for her weekly walk to the Botanical Gardens with my Aussie friend Carolyn, who was a GP. Her daughter, Georgia, was the same age as Elizabeth.

I started weeping as the little girls chased the peacocks, and when I told Carolyn not to worry about me and that I would be fine, she told me quietly but firmly to go and make an appointment at my surgery. There was something about her tone that made me feel I had better do this. Two days later I was diagnosed with severe clinical depression and put on antidepressants.

I had heard of people suffering from depression before and been rather scathing about it, imagining lazy people who couldn't be bothered to pull themselves together.

People who should really just get up and get on with it. I had been so ignorant! What I was feeling was nothing like that. I had gone beyond the dull fog that shrouded me in Hunstanton, and I was now in a state of physical panic. I told Sandy that I couldn't be more panicky if there were a T. rex behind my shoulder. I spent every weekend in bed, trying to escape from the T. rex and my mother came to the rescue again, patiently driving up the motorway from Surrey to hold the fort.

Gradually the pills started to pay dividends and first the panic, then to an extent the fog, began to dissipate. Andrew was relieved, as he had been dismayed and distressed by me being under the duvet, both literally and mentally.

Unfortunately, as the fog cleared I began to think that I could do much better without him. We had grown apart, to the point that we were co-existing but not communicating.

He went out to work as he always had done, and to me his life seemed normal. I was jealous, juggling the children and bearing all of the emotion of James's disability by proxy, as I saw it, since Andrew could rarely now come to appointments. We never talked about how it all felt.

I asked him to move out and then it was his turn to fall apart. I saw how much he loved me and how he didn't want to let me go – wouldn't let me go.

We went to marriage guidance counselling and found ourselves talking to each other as human beings and friends for the first time in five years. We discovered that each of us blamed ourselves for James's early birth, which was ridiculous as it was no one's fault.

After our third session, we sat in the pub (something we also hadn't done for five years) feeling an unaccustomed warm glow at our recovering relationship. 'The thing is, Jane,' he said, 'no one else would have either of us, because no one else would be able to deal with the poo fests!' He was quite right of course.

James had two more seizures that year and another

111

EEG, which showed for the first time evidence of epilepsy. He now had yet another diagnosis to add to the list. As one carer put it, 'A nice little package!' The impact was less than when he was diagnosed with autism however, since he had been having seizures for many months and we just wanted to stop them from happening.

The fear of finding him limp and blue after a seizure, was something that gripped my throat every morning when I went into his bedroom. If I woke in the night and he was quiet, I would be compelled to check he was ok, as he made no noise when he fitted. Even in my exhausted state, the tension prevented me from going back to sleep. I could never seem to reach a state of complete unconsciousness; never truly escape.

He was prescribed anti-fitting medication on a daily basis and also emergency medication which he had to carry around with him at all times. He was now a 'medicalised' person: it would have been criminally negligent to take him anywhere without his medication box in case he had a seizure and needed to be sedated. I began to realise that I couldn't any longer leave him at the crèche in my gym, or with the cleaning lady. I couldn't in fact leave him anywhere, unless the person he was left with could take responsibility if he fitted. We were already pretty housebound with James, now our freedom was being curtailed even further.

At the end of the year, Andrew and I sat in Dr A's office for a routine appointment while she considered James's overall health and progress. We had now known her for five years and the conversation veered on to the rest of the family, not just James. We told her about poo fests and awful holidays that were anything but holidays, and about how we had nearly divorced. She listened gravely and then said 'How old is James now, five? You've done very well to get this far without any respite breaks.'

We didn't know what respite breaks were, so we asked her. She explained that children like James could go to special units for overnight stays to give their parents a break. It would be paid for by social services.

It was as if someone had just told us there was a way out of a locked dungeon. We went home and for the first time in a very long time I felt there might be a future for us: a future that was worth living.

*

In 2004 James had three seizures and two hospital admissions.

Chapter 8
THE FIGHT BEGINS
2005

In early January of 2005, Andrew, and I sat in an office at the child development centre talking to an advocate. Dr A had referred us for some help in getting respite from social care. In normal circumstances we would have been more than capable of doing this ourselves. However, we had never had anything to do with social care before, so this was new territory. We were also so low in spirits that we were only too glad when someone offered to do it for us. We had surrendered ourselves to a system. We felt as powerless as children.

The advocate interviewed us and then sent us a letter which she had prepared, based on what we had said. That letter was to the disabled children's team at Birmingham City Council, setting out the family's need for respite from caring from James. It was odd to read about our own family as described by someone else. When we saw in black and white that I was on antidepressants, that our marriage was under severe strain, and that two of our children had been seen by a clinical psychologist, it was rather sobering.

A month later, our first social worker, # 1, came to the house to discuss the situation. She arrived with a pad of paper and asked us to tell her about James. We were happy to talk and told her all about the family situation. She made a lot of notes. She was doing what we later learned was called an initial assessment. We told her what Dr A had said, and that we wanted regular residential respite for James. She said she would have to go and talk to her manager. A few days later she came back. She told us that

James was considered too young for residential respite. He wouldn't be granted it until he was seven, and even then the maximum was two overnight stays per month. We could, however, apply for direct payments: this was money we could use to put him in the respite centre ourselves.

This didn't make sense to us. If they thought James was too young to go to the respite centre, why would they give us money to send him there?

But if that was the way it was to be done we wouldn't argue; all that mattered was that we had a meaningful break from caring for him.

The social worker said that there was a childminding inclusion scheme, where a carer could come to our house to look after James while we went out with the other children. We would also be referred to Barnado's for family support. The childminder sounded great. Barnado's sounded scary –wasn't that a charity for waifs and strays? The social worker left.

We hadn't heard anything from her by the Easter holidays, so I booked James into a play scheme run by a children's charity at the child development centre. He could go there for a few hours each day, for one week. I brought a full note telling the staff how to handle him, his emergency epilepsy medication, and a packed lunch containing foods that I knew he would eat. The children who went to the play scheme weren't all physically disabled, and so I checked there would be a member of staff allocated to look out just for James.

Two hours later I got a phone call from the centre manager. 'Er, there's been a bit of an accident. Some of the children went out to a local playground, James was put on a roundabout in his wheelchair and it fell off. We've had the doctor out and he doesn't think James has broken his nose.'

I had dealt with so much trauma that when news of a fresh one arrived, I didn't react as I would have done a few years earlier. The surge of adrenaline just wasn't there. Instead there was that cold dull feeling.

I got to the centre and found James sitting in his wheelchair, looking very white and tearful, with vivid pink scratches and bruises over his nose and mouth. The headrest of his wheelchair, which was held in place with a thick steel bar, had been knocked with such force that it was now pointing backwards rather than upwards. It wasn't a standard wheelchair either – this was specially made, and very strong.

Even the metal plates on which his feet were strapped were now buckled. I thought of how he must have felt, hurtling to the ground face first, strapped into his heavy chair like a trussed chicken. He wouldn't even have been able to put both arms out to save himself, as he couldn't move his left arm.

If it weren't for the depression I would have been spitting with rage, however I was still far from functioning normally. I didn't have the energy to spit with rage. So I took James to A&E at City Hospital to get him thoroughly checked over. Then I took him home, singing ditties to him all the way and driving with one hand so that I could hold his right hand with the other. For the next week he was very subdued and the pink scratches turned into blue bruises and then yellow patches.

I brought a personal injury claim on James's behalf, which was settled six years later. During the case, James was examined by a psychiatrist who diagnosed post-traumatic stress disorder as a result of the accident. My poor, poor James. For a while I didn't trust anyone to look after him, and I was very low, thinking that no one except me and a couple of special individuals could ever take care of him.

I wouldn't have gone near that charity again, so their play scheme was out of the question. The nursery with the cuddly girl was only available in the summer. Andrew and I were desperate to get James started at the respite centre, so we decided to go and visit it.

The Norman Laud Centre was about half an hour away,

in a north Birmingham suburb. As we approached the door we noticed that there were security gates on the windows and two coded doors to get through before you were inside. The front was bright and welcoming, with 'Hello' spelt out in yellow in about 20 different languages – appropriate for multicultural Birmingham.

We were given a professional tour of the Centre, which was a charity, not part of the local authority. We discovered that an overnight stay cost £120. Even for us, that made any regular respite prohibitively expensive. They told us that they took children from as young as 18 months. We went into the main lounge where there were several children watching TV. Although I was used to James and the other children at his school, I was still taken aback.

The children in the lounge had a much broader range of disabilities than I had experienced before, and I found myself disturbed by them.

Most of the children were able to walk, and several had challenging behaviours. One child shouted continually. Another large teenage boy was very tactile and kept trying to hug me, which I found disconcerting.

The staff were wonderful. I was very searching in my questions and eagle-eyed with what I saw, as I no longer took at face value the ability of any organisation to care safely for James. I had been let down by two children's charities already. Before the roundabout incident a carer from another charity had sat him on a kitchen chair which he nearly fell off. But I decided I would be happy to let him stay at Norman Laud.

At the end of the Easter holiday, the social worker visited us again. This time she had two other people with her. They sat in our living room and asked us how we were. We told them the truth and Andrew broke down in tears as he once again described our daily lives.

The visitors looked on sorrowfully, and one of them said that James should be 'accommodated' for a few months to give us a chance to recover. We had no idea what he meant, so he explained that James could go and stay with another family while we recovered for a while. We really were very low at that point and unable to think clearly, but I do remember my incredulity at anyone suggesting that our son should go and live with another family.

Then the social worker told us that we weren't after all going to be given money to send James to the Norman Laud Centre because he was too young. He needed to be seven, she said. Though this did make more sense than what she had previously said about direct payments, it also meant we wouldn't get any respite from James at all.

We didn't understand: the advocate at the child development centre had said we should qualify as top priority for respite. The social worker had said three months earlier that we *would* get money for respite. Now we were being told that it would be another two years (until James was seven) before we got *any* respite from anywhere.

Suddenly the way out of the dungeon that we had glimpsed – that tiny speck of light which had begun to seem nearer and nearer and to grow into a ray – had been snuffed out again. Andrew and I could not have been more devastated and deflated.

In angry desperation, I challenged the social worker. I pointed out that we had visited the Norman Laud Centre and that the staff there were happy to take children from 18 months old. I also told her that we knew a five-year-old boy was being funded by the Council to be there. But she was embarrassed and, as a junior in her department, unauthorised to change the decision that had been made by her manager.

I asked about the other help she had mentioned at the meeting three months earlier. One of the people with her was a representative from Barnado's, who had come to offer family support. We agreed that he would play football in the garden with Tom after school, on the days when James's therapists were visiting, to give him some one-to-one interaction.

Finally, there was the childminding scheme. The social worker opened her briefcase and gave us a leaflet. After she had gone, I looked at it and saw that although she had previously said that the childminder would come to us, in fact James would have to go to the childminder's house. I couldn't see this working as James with his autism would hate the strange house, and I wondered how they would find someone specialised enough to look after him.

After the social worker had gone, I registered for the childminding scheme anyway and rang them up periodically, but they never found anyone who could look after James.

I wasn't going to give up. I appealed, setting out why James should be given time at the Norman Laud Centre and how the decision not to grant it was unsupportable. It took three months to get a response. Then the social worker rang to say she wanted to come and see me. We arranged a date but she didn't turn up.

Ten days later I received a phone call from a manager at the disabled children's team. I made a note of what she said although I didn't understand it. The gist of my note was that the initial assessment carried out by the social worker in February was out of date, so the request for respite had been refused by a panel.

When I did eventually meet up with the social worker, she was very unhappy at the system she was working under and made a point of telling me this, so that I could understand why things just weren't happening. The social worker said she would need to do another initial assessment, but she thought she could do it based on the previous papers to speed things up. We arranged to meet two weeks later for me to sign it.

A month after that, the social worker called to say that we had been granted 24 nights per year for James at the Norman Laud Centre. We would also be given £1,000 towards domiciliary care and specialist toys. We hadn't asked for the one-off payment but we were exhilarated when we heard the news about the respite. It was such a tiny amount, but we had waited so long for it that it would be like drops of honey to a starving man.

James had his first visit to the Norman Laud Centre in December. Afterwards, I reflected that our family had approached the disabled children's team of Birmingham City Council in January. We had been told by the advocate at the child development centre that we were a family in crisis – a top priority for respite care – yet it had taken 10 months and an appeal to get it.

That year another woman killed her disabled son and then tried to kill herself. Wendolyn Markcrow had cared for her son with Down's syndrome for 36 years. One night she gave him 14 sleeping tablets and suffocated him with a plastic bag over his head. She then tried to cut her own throat. The son had weighed 16 st and hit himself repeatedly around the head. He also hit his parents. He had disturbed sleeping patterns and only slept for 2-3 hours each night.[6]

I didn't hear of the case at the time, but in later years it added to my deep unease at the lack of support for the parents of disabled children. How could devoted mothers, the kind you would imagine buying the weekly groceries and doing homework with their children, end up killing them?

After yet another poo fest, I decided we really had to do something to stop James getting into his pad. We were OK most of the time when he was downstairs, as long as we kept checking him regularly for any scent of an impending bowel movement. Nights were more of a problem, when he woke up and bounced unattended. The school staff didn't know of any special garments and at that time I couldn't find anything on the internet. I surfed for hours with no luck. Eventually I decided I was going to have to design something myself and get it made. I came up with

[6] *Sandra Laville, The Guardian, 3 November 2005.*

a garment that looked like a Victorian man's bathing suit. It was sleeveless and had short legs that stopped just above the knee.

It fastened at the back rather than the front, to deter James's inquisitive hands. I found a dancewear shop that would make it in a comfortable cotton/lycra mix, and within a few weeks we had our first poo-proof garments.

For a few months, until James worked out how to get into them, life was considerably sweeter.

That year, Rachel's mother Fiona, from conductive education, who had become a good friend of mine, held a party for Rachel in her garden. I thought how brave she was. The most I had been able to bring myself to do for James's birthday was to have a family tea, and even that had been traumatic. James had been unused to so much noise and fuss. We had put a tape of children's party songs on and he had begun to retch, before we had even put our left feet in and our left feet out to the hokey cokey song.

Fiona had invited the mothers she knew from the places where she took Rachel, so naturally all the children were disabled. It was an unusual gathering but James's behaviour was the most unusual of all. He was very unhappy about going to this strange house and began wailing and rocking in his wheelchair when we pulled up outside.

I had hoped that being in a disabled environment would make him feel comfortable, but not a bit of it. I took him into the garden and helped him down out of his wheelchair onto the grass. He crawled straight to the French windows and began banging his head against them so hard that I was afraid they would crack. I put him back in his wheelchair, and took him inside in front of the TV.

Fiona put on *Tweenies*, one of his minor favourites but still one he would listen to. However, he bucked continuously so hard in his chair that I thought he would tip himself over, despite the stabilisers on the back. I had been there for all of 20 minutes when I gave up and took James home. Fiona would later tell me how she had never seen a child behave like that before and it had shocked even her.

On Christmas Eve, we took James to an early service at church, the Lighting of the Lamps. It was a short service focused on small children and had always worked with James, because it contained a lot of well-known carols. He loved music, and would rock happily in his chair as everyone sang and the organ boomed. This time, however, he was in an impish mood, eating the service sheet, throwing the hymn books on the floor and demanding food endlessly, in return for a few seconds of stillness. The church was packed and I had to sit with him clamped in a bear hug to stop him pinching the children around us. I didn't mind as he kept playing with my hair and giving me dribbly kisses.

A few weeks later I was sitting in Carolyn's kitchen. Our little girls were playing around our feet while we had snatches of grown-up conversation.

Carolyn's daughter Georgia had a party whistle, which shot out a long red paper tongue. She stood next to us making a hooting noise with the whistle, the paper tongue going out and in, out and in, right next to our ears.

She was laughing with the spontaneous joy of small children tickled by a simple thing, and her laughter was so infectious that we all joined in. For Carolyn and me it was also funny because the red paper tube inflating and deflating reminded us inescapably of something else. It was so good to laugh for a long time, right from the bottom of my belly. It was an unfamiliar feeling.

The girls disappeared upstairs and Carolyn picked up her coffee looking thoughtful. 'I feel … as if I owe you an apology' she said. 'I've always seen Jamie as just a bunch of medical problems, but when I saw you with him in church, I realised that he's your child and you love him just as much as you love your other children and he's suffering.' I felt an intense emotion, pretty much love, for my friend.

In 2005 I stopped counting James's hospital admissions and seizures. The number didn't seem to matter any more.

What did seem increasingly to matter was the service we were now receiving from the Council. I didn't know it then, but an annual report on this service was produced. This year it was by both Ofsted and the Commission for Social Care Inspection.

*

The annual performance assessment of Birmingham City Council's education and children's social care services 2005 found:

'Areas for improvement ...
• *development of services for children with disabilities.'*[7]

---

[7] *Annual performance assessment of Birmingham City Council's education and children's social care services 2005. Ofsted/Commission for Social Care Inspection, 1 December 2005.*

Chapter 9
THE RESERVOIR BECKONS
2006

By early 2006, we had put James into the Norman Laud Centre for a few experimental overnight stays. However, the time came when we wanted to take a break away from Birmingham without him, a real break, something that we hadn't ever been able to do. We booked a three-day trip to London. It was so important to us, such a life-changing event, that even when we realised that the date clashed with Andrew's mother's 70th birthday party, we still decided to go. It was not an easy decision, but was helped by the fact that we knew that Babcia understood. A Polish refugee at the age of five, fleeing Stalin and Hitler, she was no stranger to suffering. It was sobering to find that she regarded our situation as very serious.

When we got on the train to go south, I had a physical feeling of release. I was able to relax in a way that I hadn't done since James was born. I knew he was in good hands and I wasn't going to be responsible for him for three whole days. Even if he had a fit, someone else would give him his medication and hold him while he recovered. The relief was indescribable. All of us felt it.

On the first day, we were like baby moles that had come up out of the ground. We were seeing the sun for the first time and were fumbling around and blinking. It felt that unreal. We went on a boat trip up the Thames and were able to listen to the guide telling us about the gruesome heads outside the Tower of London on Traitors' Gate in bygone days. He pointed out the ark-shaped building that housed the Mayor of London's headquarters, and he joked that various governments had wished they had the power to revive the tradition of beheading political rivals.

We didn't have to worry if James would try to dive over the side of the boat, or would go berserk, or would need his pad changing in the middle of the ride. We could relax and be normal.

On the second day we were totally exuberant. We wandered along the South Bank, past St Thomas' hospital and Lambeth Palace, up to the Royal Festival Hall and the London Eye. Clowns juggled balls as we passed and frozen statues made Elizabeth gasp by coming to life all of a sudden. We ate lunch at Borough Market, paralysed by choice for a while between genuine Spanish tapas, hot French lamb baguettes or Turkish meze. On the third day, we woke up, realised we had to go and pick up James, and our brief taste of freedom ended.

In some ways, it was more difficult to deal with than if we had never had the break at all. Fire-fighting had become a way of life and in its simplicity it was easy. Andrew and I had little choice about the way we spent our days, from the minute we woke up until almost the minute we went to sleep. Now we had tasted sweet freedom and were quivering with the reawakening of the memory of a previous life, which we had sublimated. The other children were coming alive with something they had never known. It was at once too much and too little.

*

For a few years now we had been trying to keep James as independent as possible, by leaving him out of his wheelchair when he was at home. We had taught him to slide safely down the stairs feet first on his stomach, although he would tease us by turning around on the half landing and pretending that he was going to launch head first. He loved to laugh at our panic-stricken faces. He was careful, however, and didn't put himself in physical danger.

When he got to the bottom of the stairs he would crawl into the playroom.

He could pull himself up onto a low bench to watch his videos and get down from it again safely if he was hungry, to crawl into the kitchen. He wouldn't go into any other room, though. It was as if the thresholds of the other rooms held untold horrors for him, and he stuck to his normal routes as if they were tramlines.

Sometimes we would 'walk' him into the kitchen for meals, standing behind him holding him under the arms. He could take steps and bear his own weight when we did that. The one thing he couldn't do was to get upstairs. He had to be carried, and there came a point where we could see that this wasn't going to change. He would only get bigger and heavier, so we were going to have to bite the bullet and get a lift.

We knew from the occupational therapist that a stairlift that whizzed up the banisters wouldn't work for James. He needed to be able to go upstairs in his wheelchair, so we were looking at a domestic version of the lifts in department stores, which would cost about £10,000.

I found that there were only four companies that put in through-floor domestic lifts, and I had all of them round to quote. The through-floor lift industry seemed to attract a particular type of rep. There was no one under the age of about 50, and they were all very serious, with short hair and sober suits.

The third man who came was a bit snappier than the others. He had a DVD for me to watch, which showed a smiley lady in a pink cardigan in a wheelchair, going up and down. After the man had measured up the floor area and worked out where the joists were, he talked about how much James weighed. He hadn't realised he was only seven. I told him we had wanted a lift three years earlier, but had waited until it was absolutely necessary because of the cost. 'I shouldn't tell you this', he said 'but I think they've changed the rules. I think disabled children now get the lifts for free.' I was so delighted that my first impulse was to kiss him. However, on looking at what appeared to be Brylcreemed hair, I quickly had second thoughts and gave him a bottle of red wine instead.

I rang the occupational therapy service who confirmed that adaptation work to the houses of disabled children was no longer means tested. There was, however, a two-year waiting list.

My expression must have resembled a freeze frame from a cartoon. We had been on a waiting list, but then we had been told we didn't qualify! Our file had been shelved! No one had told us about the change in the rules! Now we would go to the back of the queue. Who could I strangle?

Fortunately our occupational therapist came to the rescue. He resurrected our old file somehow, and so we were catapulted back to our former place on the list.

The lift was ordered and a grand fitting date set. A large hole was cut into James's bedroom floor, through which the lift would pass down into the utility room. I was as excited about getting it as a child looking forward to Christmas. I told James that when he came home from school, I would have a fantastic surprise for him. But by lunchtime on the appointed day, no one had arrived.

I rang the lift company. They didn't know what was happening and told me they would ring me back. It turned out the lift was in a container from Ireland which had been lost. They said they couldn't find it and the only thing they could do was to order another one.

I now felt like a small child on Christmas Day when Father Christmas had forgotten to come. I later found out that the lift company was on a final warning from the Council for bad service, and that as a result of my case they were likely to lose their contract.

The withdrawal of means testing didn't only apply to

lifts, it meant that all fixtures were now available on the basis of need, and so we had another assessment, to plan a full adaptation of the house for James. It was a strange process. I felt very fortunate that the state was spending all this money on our child. I was aware that if James lived in Romania he might have passed his life in a cage. However, he was still only seven, and yet we had to consider the equipment he would need as a man.

Once again we had to look into the future and try to anticipate it. In the same way as the form for claiming disability living allowance had been painful, I once again had to think about how disabled James was. This time, I also had to consider how disabled he was going to be. Andrew was 6 ft 4 in tall and James was likely to be, too. Where on earth did that leave us, in ten year's time?

A senior man from the Council who authorised the money, came and took a look around. He liked our banisters, which were carved Victorian oak, and startled me a bit by saying that his colleague loved old buildings and would have orgasms if he saw them. He was helpful in working out what we needed and how much it would cost. We couldn't have an up and down bath (a pity) but even with a wet room it would cost about £22,000 (gulp).

Everything was ordered and when the lift finally did come, the whole family enjoyed riding up and down in it. James's sister was the envy of her friends, for having such a marvellous toy. James instantly worked out how to use it. There was a set of controls inside the lift and sets on the wall nearby, both upstairs and downstairs. The buttons were colour coded and James and I would have button fights. I would send him up using the blue button on the wall and once he was 3 ft up he would send himself down using the green button inside the lift. Sometimes he would press the red alarm button just for added sound effects.

We started off by keeping the lift in his room at night, so that the utility room was clear and we could carry on doing the washing. But at 4 o'clock one morning, Andrew and I were awoken by the unwelcome sound of *Teletubbies* coming from the playroom below us. Although James was barricaded in his room at night, he had crawled into the lift, sent himself down, crawled into the playroom, switched on the TV and put on a video. From then on, the lift was stowed safely downstairs at bedtime.

Having been deprived of his late-night entertainment, James decided to explore other avenues of stimulation. He had a connecting door from his bedroom to the bathroom, which we had thought was James-proof: we were wrong. One morning I came into his bedroom to find that he wasn't there. There was a little chuckle from the bathroom and I went in, my mind already racing with guilty thoughts of him drinking toilet cleaner. He was kneeling on the floor bouncing. He had managed to take the lid off the Sudocrem – a particularly sticky white ointment used for nappy rash. He had smeared it all over the floor, adding a sprinkling of talcum powder for effect. He had also been gnawing the wooden toilet seat, which looked as if it had been got at by a chipmunk. He was very pleased with himself, so I found myself unable to be cross with him.

By the end of the year the bathroom had a sliding door which really was James-proof and a wet room, courtesy of the Council. There was a shower changing table, like a nappy changing table only adult sized. It could go up and down and had a shower hose over it so I could wash James lying down. The toilets and taps had huge handles that could easily be flicked to one side. The idea was that maybe James would one day be able to use them himself. They were so much better than ordinary taps that I wondered why people didn't have them all the time.

Hoists hung from the ceiling of James's bedroom and the playroom, and we had a ramped path that led from the back door down to the street.

There was no doubt now that ours was a house where a

disabled person lived. The equipment made such a difference to our lives though, that I embraced it. There was no point trying to hide or play down James's disabilities. He was no longer easily portable and his behaviour, not so dissimilar to the average toddler when he was two, now marked him out as a very different eight-year-old to the others he met in the normal world.

Elizabeth took it all for granted, putting her dolls in the wheelchair, playing with the lift and sending herself up and down on the changing table. To her, the paraphernalia of disability was natural scenery. Tom, who had been the subject of some of James's more vicious attacks when he was younger, still kept a wide berth.

The speech and language therapist at the special school had been working hard with James, and he was now able to make sentences, using basic symbols. For example, he could place a laminated card with the words 'I want' next to a picture of the object he wanted on a Velcro board. This made a sentence. 'I want - music/a ball/Mummy.' We had tried to do this at home but all of us found it frustrating. We had our own way of understanding James, and he didn't want to use cards at home.

As usual in the winter months, James had a chest infection and this time he refused to eat for ten days. After sleepless nights trying and failing to feed him more than a few sips of water, I took him to the surgery. By now any of my children had to be at death's door before I took them to the GP. I was usually treated well and sympathetically, but on this occasion the staff had had to cope with an emergency admission, so James and I had been forgotten. After two hours of trying to soothe his anxiety at being in a strange place and he had eaten the magazines, tried to attack the nearby toddlers and gone through every scrap of food I had packed, I was gibbering.

When I finally took James into the doctor's office, I opened my mouth and nothing came out.

I was seeing one of the senior partners rather than a junior doctor, and he took stock of the situation and bravely told me that James was about to turn a corner and would get better within a couple of days. The doctor wasn't going to give me antibiotics. He invited me to come back if James didn't get better. He was, however, sufficiently moved by the state I was in to offer to prescribe any other drugs I felt I needed.

I gladly asked him for some expensive Paracetamol suppositories, which were useful when James had a seizure and couldn't keep Calpol down. Two days later, James started to eat again.

Despite being able to handle James physically with greater ease because of the new equipment in the house, handling his behaviour was getting more and more difficult. His sleeping had become worse and worse and consequently so had ours. He would often need to sleep in the day to catch up on his 4am starts. He was refusing to come into the kitchen at mealtimes, bracing himself against the bench he sat on to watch videos, when we tried to fetch him. He was too big now for me just to pick up, and he bit me if he didn't want to come. He was increasingly reluctant to go anywhere at all outside the house, particularly in the car. He wasn't really living with us but co-existing: going only in the playroom, eating different food from us at different times to us, and sleeping when we were awake. We were painfully aware that this was having a devastating effect on the other children, and Andrew and I were just limping along in survival mode.

The handling assessment form from his school for that period showed that the problem of his challenging behaviour was not confined to home.

James rocks uncontrollably in his seating system & in his standing frame. ...James tends to mouth everything & he will bite staff/children.'

131

The difference between school and home though, was that when he was at school James was meaningfully occupied by a team of people. He was also happy to go on trips on the school bus, to places he had never been before.

In April we had a letter from another social worker. Now that James was receiving respite care he was under a different team. The new social worker, # 2, came to the house to meet me.

Like her predecessor, she started by getting out her pad and pen and saying 'So tell me about James.' I obligingly went through his medical history and current abilities and disabilities.

I also told her what the family had been through. She seemed more experienced than her predecessor, and she too was sympathetic and helpful. At the time I didn't realise that she was carrying out another initial assessment. Her note of our meeting which I saw later said:

James is needs [sic] are overpowering his family and they have struggled caring for him. They feel that they are on the brink of having to put him into care but do not wish to. I feel this family needs more support and need another weekend a month of respite care and some time of home assistance.'

I don't recollect ever asking for James to be taken into care. I didn't really know at that point what 'being taken into care' meant. However, at the back of my mind I was beginning to have visions of a place where James could live, where there was always a team of people around to occupy and handle him. A place where he would be happy to go out on organised trips and would eat cooked food socially at mealtimes with everyone else.

The visions were not even fully formed in my own head, although I must have said something to social worker # 2, for her to think I was talking about James going into care.

Along with these visions of residential care, I was having

another sort of vision. The beach hut picture had lost its power, and I was now seeking refuge in dreams about walking into our local reservoir. I didn't imagine the bit between leaving home and arriving there. It was an isolated fantasy, inspired by the peace and coolness that would come from walking into water until it closed over my head and shut out the chaos around me. In my fantasy I wore a ball and chain around my ankle. I told my GP about this and he said it was called having 'suicidal thoughts'. He said that when you were stuck in an intolerable situation from which there was no way out, your mind would provide you with fantasies of one. He asked me some questions and seemed satisfied that there was still a gap between fantasy and reality, but he wanted to see me regularly to keep a close eye on me.

That year, yet another mother committed suicide with her disabled child. Alison Davies jumped off the Humber Bridge with her 12-year-old son. He had Fragile X syndrome and exhibited behavioural problems and learning difficulties.[8]

My friend Joanna later confided in me that it was only when she told her GP that she could understand why the woman had leapt off the Humber Bridge, that she and the vicar had begun to get help from social care for their autistic son, Edmund.

In May, Andrew and I went to what would be one of many reviews of James's progress, at the Norman Laud Centre. The manager there explained to me that James was now a 'looked after child' (LAC) – a statutory definition meaning he was being looked after by the Council.[9] This was because the Council was paying for his accommodation while he was at the Centre, and he was taking overnight stays. This in turn meant that an independent reviewing officer (who was nevertheless an employee of the Council) would have to review his progress every six months.[10] The officer wouldn't just be looking at the respite provision – he would officially review all aspects of James's life.

[8] Deidre Fernand, *The Sunday Times*, 21 May 2006.
[9] *Children Act 1989 section 22(1)*.
[10] *Ibid section 25A*.

I didn't like the idea of that at all. Why, when James had two devoted parents looking after him, did someone from the state need to check that he had been to the dentist, was being kept clean and was attending school? It seemed a gross invasion of our family's privacy.

I didn't know at the time that most looked after children were in foster care. The system was geared up to children who didn't live with their natural parents, due to difficulties at home. In 2010 only 3 per cent of children were looked after because they were disabled.[11]

When we arrived for our first LAC review, social worker # 2 was there, together with the head of the Norman Laud Centre. The independent reviewing officer wanted to hear the full story about James. I told him about the history of our attempts to get respite and the current state of the family. He became very grave.

This is what he minuted afterwards:

'After considerable discussion at review the Reviewing Officer was not clear as to ... why this family who are caring for a severely disabled child and have done so from birth have had such difficulties being assessed for respite, nor why James is now seven years old and has only had involvement with the Social Services via assessment since the end of 2005. The answers to these questions were not available at review nor perhaps are there answers available to some of the questions but the Reviewing Officer asked that [the social worker] attempt to establish from the files and from previous workers why this situation has arisen in this manner for the family and why so many appeals have been necessary.'

Until I read this I had had no idea that we were supposed to have been supported by social care since James's birth. I later found out that disabled children are automatically defined as 'children in need' under the Children Act 1989. The Council

11 *Department for Education Statistical First Release SFR21/2011 28 September 2011, Children looked after in England (including adoption and care leavers) year ending 31 March 2011.*

had a statutory duty to safeguard and promote his welfare, by providing a range and level of services appropriate to his needs.[12] James had been a child in need since birth, but we had not received any support until he was seven.

It was nice to have the independent reviewing officer being indignant on our behalf. Perhaps this review business wasn't so bad after all.

By July social worker # 2 had obtained funding for more respite care. We now had five nights per month, which made a total of 60 nights per year.

She told me that it was a very large package. She also obtained for us £256 to buy a special jumbo-sized remote control from the US. It had buttons the size of golf balls and would allow James to wind his *Teletubbies* tapes back and forth, without wrecking the video player. We knew that videos were becoming obsolete and it was getting harder and harder to replace his favourites.

We used to trawl the local charity shops looking for second-hand ones. We didn't like to think about what we would do when even this source dried up. If we converted to DVDs it would cost us a fortune, as James would bite them and ruin them within hours.

When the school broke up for the summer holiday, we had a panic about James's pads. The nurses at school usually ordered them, and they were delivered in bulk to our front door once every few months. On this occasion, the delivery company swore they had delivered them and I swore that they hadn't.

There was a stand-off and then it came to the last day of term. I was facing a six-week holiday with no pads for an incontinent child. It didn't occur to me to buy some myself. This was probably because James was much too big for even the biggest products I could get from the supermarket, and it didn't occur to me to look for specialist suppliers online. I was in the fog of depression. I could only think in straight lines, because it was easier and a question of surviving. If I

---

[12] *Children Act 1989 section 17(1)(a).*

followed the straight lines, I could get to the end of each day.

On this occasion I went into school to beg the nurses to intervene. They went into overdrive and by the time I got home, there was another pallet of pads on the doorstep. Phew!

The children having broken up, there was the usual issue of what on earth to do with all of them. Tom was then nine, James was seven and Elizabeth was three. James would have a week with his cuddly girl at the nursery for deprived children, and we now had extra respite, so we could take a family holiday without him. There were still all the other days to fill. I planned some things and took the rest of it on a day by day basis.

One of the planned things was a joint trip to Twycross Zoo with Carolyn and her kids. I had high hopes for this outing. Our daughters were good friends. Tom was younger than Carolyn's son, but we thought they would get along. I was sure James would be fascinated by the animals.

When we got there, the other children did get on, but as for James enjoying the animals, not a bit of it. He was bored rigid by the giraffes, the lions and the hippopotamuses. When we went to the play area he became very distressed, and I had to put his coat over his head so that he was 'blacked out'. This meant that he could go to sleep, which is what he needed, but passers-by looked on in concern and astonishment, thinking I was inflicting some strange punishment. Carolyn and I stood on piles of bark chippings watching the little girls play on the swings, while James rocked himself to sleep in his wheelchair, looking like a demented black ghost.

On the days in the holidays when I hadn't planned anything, I tried to take James out as little as possible, as it was such a fraught process and almost inevitably ended up with him attacking someone. The school summer holiday was so long though, that after a while I would become stir crazy.

I felt as if I were stuck in Groundhog Day – trapped in a predictable routine carried out in the same way, in the same place each day, without any variation. After a few days of being stuck in the house, the lure of seeing anything that wasn't the four walls of the kitchen would become too much and I would pack the children into the car and set off. It took about an hour to go, because everyone had to have been recently fed and toileted. Also, to get a wheelchair clamped into an adapted vehicle (which we had now bought) was a lengthy and tedious process. The four wheels of the wheelchair had to be clamped to brackets in the floor, each with their own mini seat belts. Then a mega seat belt had to be fixed over the wheelchair and James. The process had to be reversed at the other end when disembarking and then repeated on the way home.

I had tried going out for walks instead of using the car, but the streets of the neighbourhood we lived in weren't always very nice. Sometimes we had to avoid piles of litter and used condoms. The Botanical Gardens, which was only half a mile away, was a place that James now refused to go to, so it was out of the question. There was the local reservoir, also just around the corner. However, the last time I had tried to take James there, he had thrown a tantrum because I had forgotten to take food with me. I had become so desperate at his behaviour that I had knocked at the vicarage door, which was on the way, and asked Joanna for something to eat – like a destitute character from a Dickens novel. Fortunately the vicarage was a sympathetic place for me and some bread was gladly forthcoming, which calmed James down.

In the middle of that summer, I realised that my mother's birthday was coming up and I didn't have a card. Since I could never repay her for all the support and love she had given us, I wasn't going to miss it. So an hour later, we all stood in Clinton Cards in our local high street. James hadn't wanted to go out at all, and once we entered the shop he went crazy.

I had a full-scale tantrum on my hands: he was wailing, flailing his arms and rocking so hard I thought he would tip his industrial strength wheelchair over. He hit his own head and bit his hand. I tried to calm him by talking gently and hugging him but I was rewarded with a bite and a slap. I had had all the children off school for several weeks and was very very weary. Tears began to form in my eyes as I withdrew from James for a minute to try to choose a card, any card, so that we could leave. The idea of going home without the card was unthinkable. All that effort for nothing!

James's behaviour was making everyone both inside and outside the shop stop and stare at him in disbelief. But out of the corner of my eye I noticed a woman who was looking at me in a different way from all the others. She wasn't shocked at what she was seeing, she was sympathetic. She was hovering at the edge of the situation, wondering what to do. Then she walked away to the counter. I managed to grab a card for my mother and I went up to the counter too. The woman turned around with her purchase and gave it to me. 'This is for you, you are doing a wonderful job', she said. I took the bag she had given me and opened it. Inside was the thing she had just bought. It was a tiny teddy wearing a lilac T-shirt which said: 'World's no. 1 Mum!'

That was another golden nugget to be stored in my treasure chest, just like the comment of the lady who had done James's first EEG and told me she could see that I had made a difference with all the therapies.

That summer, Andrew told me that there was no future for his type of work in the Midlands. 'I'm going to have to move my career to London', he said. 'That is where it's all happening. If I stay here I'll be out of a job.' This was very difficult to hear, particularly as my own father had emigrated to Los Angeles when I was a teenager.

I felt I was losing the most important man in my life all over again. But Andrew was the sole breadwinner – there was no way I was capable of working at that time – and we had to make sure he could support us. I had read of families where parents of a disabled child gave up work and lived on state benefits so that they could both be carers. That was not us. We had two other children to think of.

We considered moving back to central London so we could all be together. Then I thought of trying to take James on tube trains in his wheelchair. I thought of all the neighbours and friends we had become close to and who had a special understanding of our situation. I thought of the upheaval we had gone through when the house was adapted. I thought of the effect on the other children of uprooting them after all they had already been through. We decided that we couldn't move, we were going to have to live apart during the week.

That summer we found Andrew somewhere to stay in London from Monday to Thursday, and when the children went back to school in September, I was a single mother for much of the time.

When the autumn school term began, I saw Joanna walking past the end of my drive on the way home with some of her children. We hadn't seen each other for a couple of years. We stopped for a chat and she asked how I was. 'Not brilliant, I nearly got divorced and I had a nervous breakdown. How about you?'

I think it was the depression that made me so uninhibited, but I find even now that small talk is so boring and irrelevant. Joanna and I locked gazes for quite a long time. Then she said 'It's been a bit like that for us, too.' We looked at each other, wanting to dive into a conversation. But the children were in post-school mode and needed attention. They couldn't be parties to this. 'Let's go to the pub' she suggested. 'Yes' I said. 'I'll email you.'

We were so busy with our respective families that although we started emailing each other, we didn't go to the pub together for almost three more years. But we did manage a coffee at the vicarage while I had a look through Edmund's statement of special educational needs.

He was a weekly boarder at a school for autistic children

run by the Council. Joanna wanted to make sure that when he turned 11 years old he would be able to continue as a boarder and not become a day boy, as she couldn't have coped with that. She was very concerned about Edmund becoming unmanageable when he was bigger and stronger.

She told me again of the friend who had come to visit her and left her autistic son in the car, which was rocking and bucking in the drive. The boy was now a teenager and had developed a penchant for masturbating over door handles.

We both looked at the vicarage door, where the handle was at chest height. The same thought crossed our minds: 'He'd have to get a pretty good angle to hit that!' said Joanna.

*

In October social worker # 2 came and concluded our third initial assessment in which she recorded:

'James is now setting more boundaries and testing them. He likes to play with the VCR constantly and he will press rewind after watching his favourite bit of a show and repeated [sic] it over and over. His mother explained that is the autism in him when he focuses like this…James is very selective in his likes and dislikes, he used to love going to the park…his father explained that suddenly one day he decided he didn't like it and now kicks and screams when he has to go. James also does not like eating and in the last year instead of being able to be wheeled out to sit for dinner at the table he has learned now to brace his arms and legs so he will remain in the living room. His parents admit they give into [sic] this behaviour. During the spring break they have found that they have allowed James to watch the VCR too much but they don't know how else to keep him stimulated. Family also get quit [sic] concerned because James has nothing else to do in the home.'

I didn't see this note at the time, but when I did read it some months later I was angry at the implication that Andrew and I couldn't be bothered to discipline James's behaviour. I wondered how the social worker would have coped if she were me.

In the autumn, James had another round of Botox injections. The consultant had decided that it would be better to get him into an operating theatre this time, rather than to treat him in his bed, when he administered injections deep into his muscles. I also thought this was a good idea at the time, but the day that ensued was the worst hospital day I ever had since James had been discharged from the neonatal unit.

Firstly, James had to go to a different hospital for the procedure this time. It was the one with the Portakabins and the maze of corridors. He had to be there for 7.30am and be nil by mouth since the previous night. But this hospital was further away than the one he had been to before, so the logistics were severe. I had to ask kind neighbours to take Tom and Elizabeth in at the ungodly hour of 7.15am, which was the earliest I thought was within the bounds of decency.

Even then, I couldn't possibly get James to the hospital by 7.30am, so I had to get the staff to agree that we could turn up half an hour late. I did after all have to clamp and de-clamp James's wheelchair from the car and get him through the Portakabins. I even went through a trial run, going to the hospital the week before to see whether the disabled parking was all taken up (it was and not always by people with a Blue Badge), and working out exactly where the ward was.

Nevertheless, on the day we arrived on time, with James's siblings safely deposited with the very kind neighbours and James nil by mouth. Then there was another hurdle: I had asked for a cot rather than a bed, which was there, but this wasn't a specialised children's ward like the last one. They didn't have lots of TVs and lots of children's films. It took a long time to get a TV arranged, by which time James was climbing the bars of his cot with frustration, thirst, hunger and distress. The eventual arrival of the TV with a DVD player had the same impact on me as if the Angel Gabriel had appeared. It would have all been fine then, if James had had his surgery in mid-morning. But the hours went by and no consultant arrived. I spent every second soothing him.

As midday approached, I began to get panicky. I had to collect Elizabeth from nursery at 3pm and James hadn't even had surgery yet. I went to have a word with the nurses. They explained that the consultant had to go to a meeting at another hospital at noon, which was why he was late. The cold dull feeling came over me. Surely the consultant must have known the day before that he had a meeting? Why couldn't someone have contacted us, to say we didn't need to get here for 7.30am? Had they the faintest inkling of what I had gone through and was now still going through, to get a physically disabled, autistic child to cope with the hours in this environment without eating and drinking?

Whether what I said had any effect, or whether the consultant would have come anyway, I don't know. The nurses assured me that I would be able to leave in time to pick up my other children, then suddenly there was the consultant, James's legs were being marked up in biro, and they were taking him for his anaesthetic.

They were checking with me that James had indeed not eaten or drunk anything since 12am the night before, when I saw his mouth working. I was used to this. 'James,' I said sternly, 'give it to me!' He opened his mouth and there was the plastic tab off an ampoule of medication. He must have picked it up from somewhere in the ward when no one was looking.

The staff there wouldn't have known that he had it in his mouth, and yet he was about to be put to sleep! I wondered what would have happened if the tab had gone into his lungs while he was unconscious. Then the anaesthetist came. He was very jolly. He was probably trying to make me feel relaxed but he failed spectacularly. 'We're going to use a special drug to put James to sleep,' he said, or words to that effect. 'It's better than a general anaesthetic because we only need him to be "out" for a few minutes. We just slow his heart down so it beats very slowly. Don't worry,' he chuckled, 'we usually get it going again!'

The procedure didn't take long, but I sat outside the operating theatre in emotional agony, with a graphic image in my mind of James's heart beating slower and slower until it finally stopped. The world started again for me when he was wheeled out of theatre and eventually opened his eyes. He came round quite quickly, and I fed him a packed lunch as soon as the staff would let me. I got home just in time to pick up Elizabeth and Tom.

The next day James was completely immobilised by the newly administered Botox. The effect would gradually wear off over the next few months, but he was so disconcerted by not being able to crawl around that I wondered how useful it actually was. I was trying to make a rational argument for stopping the Botox treatment because I didn't think I could bear another hospital appointment like that.

The Christmas holidays arrived, the time I dreaded most. I had over two weeks with all three children at home, very little opportunity to get out of the house and Christmas to prepare for. For several years after James was born I didn't send any Christmas cards at all and Christmas dinner came straight from the supermarket. I had always made a point of getting stockings for the children though, including James. He was completely uninterested in toys, so had it not been for Tom and Elizabeth, I wouldn't have bought him anything. However, I knew that they wouldn't understand if Father Christmas visited them and not their brother. James's presents lay largely unopened in the playroom as he ignored them in favour of *Teletubbies*, even when we tried to sit with him to open them.

This year, his lack of interest in his presents was all the more poignant because he was becoming bored with his videos. He wouldn't look at any new stories, sticking rigidly to *Teletubbies*, with the odd foray into *Postman Pat, Fireman Sam* and *Tweenies*. He knew every inch of every tape and there was no stimulation or surprise in any of them. Despite being bored, he wouldn't countenance anything new, nor would he go out anywhere, so he was trapped watching old favourites in a prison of his own making.

I desperately wanted him to join us for lunch on Christmas Day. I tried taking him into the kitchen before everyone else so that he wouldn't be overwhelmed, and I had his food waiting there for him. It made no difference. He spent hours on Christmas Day in front of the TV in the playroom, winding and rewinding his favourite scenes, while we ate apart from him.

It was a disjointed meal because he was so bored with his tapes that he wanted to change them every ten minutes or so. However, one of us had to do that for him, as we had put the video player out of reach so he couldn't damage it, and he was using his American remote control with the massive buttons.

After a while I realised it was ominously silent and went in to find that James had abandoned *Teletubbies* and decided to feast on a slug which had made its way in through a gap in the floorboards.

He had bitten its head off and was squeezing the innards out like a tube of toothpaste, chuckling all the while. I couldn't stand the sight of it and fled, leaving Andrew to deal with the gruesome scene.

*

In 2006 a review took place of the Council's services for children and young people. This had been carried out by 11 inspectors from bodies including Ofsted, the Commission for Social Care Inspection, the Healthcare Commission and the Audit Commission. The review said:

'23. ...there is insufficient integrated assessment and coordination of services for children who have learning difficulties and/or disabilities...

'91. ...the city council took the difficult decision to postpone improving services to children with learning difficulties and/ or disabilities while it focused on improving frontline child protection and looked after children services.' [13]

[13] *Joint area review, Birmingham Children's Services Authority Area, Review of services for children and young people, Ofsted et al, carried out 2006, published 6 February 2007. (No annual performance assessment was published in 2006.)*

Chapter 10
A BIG DECISION
2007

'I have had worse partings, but none that so
Gnaws at my mind still. Perhaps it is roughly
Saying what God alone could perfectly show –
How selfhood begins with a walking away,
And love is proved in the letting go'. [14]

In the New Year, Elizabeth was invited to a party by one of her
friends from school. It was held in a barn with a soft play area,
nets to climb and a long blue slide. My lawyer friend Helen was
there with her daughter Alice, and we sat and had coffee while
the girls ran about shrieking. I felt lower at that point than I
had ever been, and I sat and wept while Helen held my hand
and stroked it, as if I were one of her children. 'My life isn't
worth living', I said, and I meant it. I saw no hope, no change,
no liberty and no sleep: just a lifetime of looking after James.

One evening the following week, I sat alone in the living
room. The children were all in bed. I wept again, and
this time something happened. My heart had recognised
something that my head didn't want to think about. James
couldn't carry on living with us. It was destroying us all. 'Oh
my baby, oh my baby', I said out loud.

My earlier vision of a residential environment, where
James could be cared for by a team of people and enjoy a
normal life going outside to different places, now hovered
in my mind. I hadn't given it a name, but it was somewhere
he would live all the time, where everything was done
to a schedule. Only if he were living in an institutional

[14] *Excerpt from 'Walking Away' by C. Day-Lewis, taken from*
his Selected Poems. Published by Enitharmon Press.

environment could he function. Only if he were living in such a place, could he cope with the changes involved with going outside.

Only if there were a team of people looking after him could we cope.

I called social worker # 2 a couple of times but missed her, so in late January I wrote her a letter, attaching a report about what life was really like for us all.

The report was called 'Life with James' and it was ten pages long. It set out all the reasons why we couldn't cope with James living at home, and how he couldn't cope with living with us.

I talked of how he attacked Tom and Elizabeth if we tried to go out in the car. I talked of how social life was impossible. I talked of poo fests. I explained how distraught I was that we couldn't occupy him meaningfully and how he was suffering. The report ended with the statement that I was depressed and sleep deprived, and that I didn't have a life.

Nothing happened.

I called soon after I sent my report, only to be told social worker # 2 was off sick. I rang again a few days later and was told she was still off sick. I was offered a call from the duty social worker, to which I said 'Yes please'. No one rang me back. Six weeks after I sent the report, I wrote to social worker # 2 again, mentioning that I hadn't heard from her. I pointed out that there was a LAC review coming up. By this stage, the place James needed to be had evolved in my mind as a residential school.

I told her I had sent a copy of my report to the independent reviewing officer and would be raising the issue of residential schooling for James at the review. Before the review, she got in touch and came to see me.

She sat in my living room, on the same chair where I had cried two months earlier. She told me that if a residential school was what I wanted, then I would have to change James's statement of special educational needs and it would be a long process. This just didn't sink in. I was too deep in fog.

Considerable confusion followed at the LAC review, as a result of my failure to understand what she had said.

I didn't realise that the disabled children's team of which she was part, was purely a social care team. In order to change James's statement of special educational needs I should have gone to the education department of the Council. At the time I didn't know that.

At the LAC review, held at the Norman Laud Centre, I explained to the independent reviewing officer that the 60 nights of respite James had at the Centre was not nearly enough. I gave her a schedule I had prepared, showing the hours of help we needed every weekend and all through the school holidays. I broke down continually.

The independent reviewing officer looked at me in alarm and concern. 'This child should be accommodated', she said. What she meant was that James should be taken into the care of the local authority. Not against my wishes – that would only have happened if I had abused or neglected him – but on a voluntary basis. She thought I was asking for James to be taken into care.

But I wasn't asking for James to be taken into care. If I had been asking for that, he might have been put with foster parents or in a children's home, while he continued to go to his Birmingham day school. I wouldn't have considered either of these options for James. He needed a residential school where his life was seamless.

I needn't have worried about James being taken into care, voluntarily or otherwise. Another social worker, # 3, who was also present at the review, told the independent reviewing officer that she had discussed the idea of 'accommodating' James with her manager and had been told it wasn't an option.

So, even if I had wanted James to be taken into care at that meeting, simply because I couldn't cope, they would have said no. That meant no foster parents, no children's home and no residential school, because that was a matter for the education department so it wasn't even considered.

Then the social worker said that James missed his family when he was away at the Norman Laud Centre. His teachers had reported that he was unsettled at school the day after he returned. On hearing this evidence of James's attachment to us, I broke down. How could I seek to have him live away from us?

The independent reviewing officer said that having more help at home might work. I was feeling so low that I had no fight left in me, so I agreed. She ordered the next review to be in just three month's time, rather than the usual six months. In the meantime, social worker # 3 undertook to carry out another initial assessment of the family within two weeks and to investigate providing some help at home.

Nothing happened.

By May James had been referred to an educational psychologist, as he had developed some challenging behaviours at school, and they wanted a strategy to cope.

I went to the school to have a chat, and ended up having a cup of tea with the head teacher, whom I liked very much. I told her how I thought James should be in a residential school and she was surprised. 'But he's so young!' she said. 'And you would be taking him away from his family!'

I was terribly upset that she of all people took this view, since I had sent her the 'Life with James' report that I had also sent to the social care department.

How could she not see that our situation was impossible? Nevertheless, I asked whether she knew of any such places where James could go.

She said that if James was to go to a residential school,

I would have to show that he needed a 'waking curriculum'. That meant that his education needed to continue beyond the normal school day. I would have to get his statement of special educational needs amended. I exclaimed, 'But that is exactly what he needs! A school like this one, but with beds!'

She was clearly unhappy with what I was saying, but I now understood the way forward. I was going nowhere with the disabled children's team, which was a social care team. I had to concentrate on James's education.

After I had left the head teacher's office, I went to see the speech and language therapist.

It was the same woman who had introduced James to PECS a few years earlier, getting him to hand her an empty packet of crisps as a 'picture' to request what he wanted. I told her my idea for a residential school and she became excited. 'That's just what he needs', she mused. 'It would be brilliant for him.' She was a great antidote to the head teacher, and once again, in her I felt I had an ally. I could see I was going to need all the support I could get.

I went home with a mission. The next day, I visited Waterstone's and went to the education section. There was a book on special educational needs and also a directory of all the special schools in the UK, the Gabbitas guide.[15] I went home and started to read.

It had been a long time since I had used my brain in any serious intellectual activity. However, after a couple of days the rust was beginning to fly off the cogs, and I was deeply engrossed.

Encouragingly, it seemed that for a disabled child, learning to walk and 'talk' could be educational needs. However, it was also the case that James's non-educational needs and any needs of the rest of the family were irrelevant. Well, at least I now knew where we stood. I read on.

If the local authority wouldn't agree that the child needed a residential school, then the parent could take the

[15] *Schools for Special Needs, Gabbitas Educational Consultants*
© *Gabbitas and Kogan Page, 2011.*

matter to an independent tribunal. I was elated: a tribunal was a legal forum, so I would be on home territory!

I would have to challenge James's statement of special educational needs. That was the piece of paper I had received five years earlier and filed without reading it. I had to get it changed so that it described his need for a waking curriculum and named a residential school. There were limited opportunities to change the statement. One was if it had been amended within the last two months. Then I had an automatic right to appeal it.

Something stirred in the depths of my memory. I had never read the statement, but hadn't I seen something like it in the post a few weeks ago? Where was it? I dug around frantically in the piles of unfiled, unanswered paperwork that lay on the floor. There were lots of things I looked for that I never found, transported by some mysterious paper goblin. However, this time I did find what I was looking for.

It was James's statement of special educational needs and it had been amended by the local authority, on a technicality. I looked at the date on it and checked my diary over and over. I only had five days left to appeal before the deadline expired.

After sitting night and day with the legal textbook, the appeal was finally lodged, and I had to turn my attention to finding the right school.

I got out the book with a list of all the special schools in the UK. There were very few local authority schools in the UK with beds. Almost all the boarding schools seemed to be independent. The schools had a list of symbols next to their names, rather like a hotel guide.

Instead of signs indicating 'high chairs available' and 'no smoking in the bedrooms', there were symbols representing the different sorts of disability catered for. So 'WA1' meant the school was fully wheelchair accessible; 'EPI' meant it catered for epilepsy; SP&LD was the symbol for speech and language difficulties.

James technically qualified for seven categories: cerebral palsy, autistic spectrum disorder, epilepsy, speech and language difficulties, severe learning difficulties, challenging behaviours, and the school must be wheelchair accessible. Seeing the extent of his disabilities listed so baldly made me catch my breath. However, I didn't want him in a school alongside children with autism or challenging behaviours who could walk, as he would be very vulnerable. I prioritised the learning and physical care he needed. I particularly wanted somewhere that offered a genuine waking day curriculum, so that he didn't have to cope with unnecessary change.

I could only find three schools in the UK that came anywhere near fitting the bill. I went to visit them. They were all over 100 miles from our home.

One school seemed to be in a state of decline. The building was rather desolate and reminded me of Thornfield Hall, in Charlotte Brontë's novel, *Jane Eyre*. I was shown around the swimming pool, without any request to remove my outdoor shoes or put shoe covers on, so any dirt I had brought in was deposited on the edge of the pool, where the residents were swimming. I dismissed that one.

The second school was livelier, but they weren't using PECS, the communication system which James had cottoned onto so successfully. A member of staff told me that she was sure she could 'get the hang of it'. That didn't fill me with confidence.

The third school was Dame Hannah Rogers School in Devon. I had been struck by their entry in the Gabbitas guide, which emphasised the seamless care provided between home and school staff.

My visit confirmed what I had read. There was a full-time nursing staff and a team of therapists employed by the school. The therapists moved between the school and the boarding wing all the time, seeing children in their bedrooms and assessing how they should be sleeping or sitting while they ate their breakfast.

The care staff would implement the therapy programmes, and follow whatever communication system each child was using. If a pupil had to ask for a banana with a hand sign at school, he (or she) also had to ask for a banana with a hand sign at bedtime.

I was particularly struck by the happy atmosphere of the place. There was a lot of teasing and joking and the staff were affectionate and respectful towards the children. The children were affectionate, if not always so respectful back!

I was interested in the fact that the school had been part of the local village for over 200 years, and so many local people worked at the school that the community was completely intertwined. The children would go to the nearby library, park, shops and church and be accepted as part of the village, without anyone batting an eyelid.

It didn't hurt that the whole complex was set in a beautiful valley, with Dartmoor rising behind it and the South Hams rolling away to the sea in front. I felt comfortable and at home, and I had no doubt that this was where James needed to be. This was what I was fighting for.

A few weeks later I took James for an official assessment there.

I had a long chat with the head teacher, and commented on how difficult it was to find out about schools like hers. I had looked into one nearer to home, but when I rang them they had said they were closing down due to falling pupil numbers.

The head teacher sighed and said that local authorities had used to send children like James to the school automatically, but now they were trying to save money by keeping them in local provision. Nowadays, she said, the only way to get a child into the school was to go to tribunal, as I was doing. I wasn't surprised, but I thought about what it meant for all the disabled children who weren't getting enough therapy where they lived. I thought of those children whose parents weren't capable, for whatever reason, of going to tribunal.

I thought of all the expertise concentrated in schools like Dame Hannah's, which were so few and far between. What a terrible waste of resources for such schools to close! What a tragedy that more children couldn't attend them! I felt it should not be allowed to happen. There should be more schools like this, not fewer.

Transporting James in the car the 200 miles to Devon was an endurance test that I wouldn't have borne for any other reason. The car we had bought which took his wheelchair was a little van for local journeys. Since we never took James far afield, it had been fine. To go 200 miles, however, I needed something which could go faster than 60mph and didn't rattle and roar at speed, so I took Andrew's car. The wheelchair had to be dismantled and would only fit in the back seat, so James had to travel next to me in the front.

He thought sitting next to Mummy was a great treat, particularly as he now had control of the radio. There were no red lights on the motorway, which was a definite plus. However, James became intrigued by the gear stick and kept trying to change gear at 90mph. As I tried to stop him, he began to attack me with his right hand, which was nearest to me. Then he discovered the steering wheel and fancied a go at driving. In the end, in order to keep us both alive, I had to strap his hand down in his seat using a luggage strap.

By the time we had arrived and were ensconced in the parents' bungalow, both of us were traumatised. First of all I set James up in front of *Teletubbies*. I had brought his jumbo remote control with the golf ball-sized buttons, and his own video player, knowing these would be needed. Once the *Teletubbies* were running around their green and pleasant land to his order, he calmed down. I then made myself a very large cup of tea.

We spent two days at the school, where they had arranged a packed assessment schedule. The physiotherapist put him in a new design of walker, which I had not seen before. After a moment of uncertainty, James began to march and then almost run down the corridor. It gave me a tearful, goose bump feeling, as I had never seen him move like that before. His face was at first absorbed with the new sensation then, as he began to move faster and faster, a broad smile crept across his face, turning finally into exhilaration.

The orthopaedic consultant asked when he had last had his hips X-rayed. I couldn't remember. (It was five years previously.) The consultant said they should be X-rayed at least every two years, since he wasn't walking. In children who didn't walk, the ball of the hip didn't get deeply embedded in the hip socket, which instead remained shallow. This in turn gave rise to a risk of dislocation. I made a mental note to ask for an X-ray when we got back to Birmingham.

The occupational therapist thought James could benefit from wearing leg gaiters at night. These were like old-fashioned girdles which went from thigh to toe, to keep his legs in a straight position while he slept and give him eight hours of stretch on his spastic muscles. I couldn't remember anyone considering his posture at night for years.

The educational psychologist was very experienced with autistic children and she understood James straight away, for which he adored her. She gave him a dark blanket which he happily put over his head for a temporary 'black out'.

After we had returned home, I received a letter from the head teacher of Dame Hannah's, offering James a placement at the school. If he went for 50 weeks (the maximum time the school was open) the annual fee would be an eye-watering £185,000. Now I just had to get the Council to pay.

One decision I had to make was whether to represent myself at the tribunal hearing, or whether to instruct another lawyer to do it for me. The tribunal was specifically designed for parents to represent themselves. It was meant to be an informal forum to avoid the necessity of legal fees.

I considered the cost of using another lawyer and for a few weeks thought that I would do it all myself. But a small part of me was scared. I was so angry with the Council and so emotional about James, I wasn't sure if I could keep my cool at the hearing. If I didn't, I could ruin James's chances.

During this time I went to my TV presenter friend Sandy's 50th birthday party. It was, not surprisingly, a glamorous event, with the hostess herself the most gorgeous in a gold silk dress. Her husband had put up an awning with coloured lights, and there were pink and purple balloons, candles, confetti and a band. I wasn't in a party mood, however. I was exhausted with all the emotion I was feeling and the constant grind of preparing paperwork for James's case. I had been deputised to take photos that night, but proved myself a bad choice. I had forgotten to check the memory card in my camera, which was malfunctioning and only held 12 photos. Worse, I stood my subjects in front of a mirror. When I viewed the pictures later, all of them had an extraterrestrial quality, as a bright ball of light hung over everyone's shoulder where the flash had bounced off the glass.

Once I had filled the memory card I spotted another lawyer friend, Harriet, and we sat on a leather couch together, drinking Mojito cocktails. I told her about the case. She leaned forward.

'Jane, don't do this on your own. Don't represent yourself. You're too involved. Get yourself a really good barrister.' I thought about the old saying 'A lawyer who represents himself has a fool for a client', and I changed my mind. So I went to a top London barrister, and the case went into top gear.

It hadn't occurred to me that we would need expert witnesses but our barrister assured me that we did, and over the next few weeks a string of professionals came to see James and to produce what I hoped would be helpful written reports.

There were speech and language therapists, occupational therapists, physiotherapists, an educational psychologist, and even an expert social worker, who was a lawyer himself. All of them worked privately for people like me. By the time the case finished, I had spent £20,000 of a cherished inheritance on them and the barrister.

*

In June, James's speech and language therapist at his Birmingham school wrote a report which was to prove pivotal at the tribunal hearing. In speech and language 'speak' she had given me, on a plate, direct evidence that James needed a waking curriculum.

She had said that the way he learned to communicate must be consistent at all times and in all environments, even at night. She said:

'...James needs an environment which:...
• Provides frequent planned opportunities to practice [sic] the targeted communication skills to promote generalisation integrated within all activities throughout the 24 hour day.'

The significance of this was immense. If we could prove that James needed a waking curriculum we could win our case at tribunal. She was his current therapist, who had known him for four years. If she was prepared to say he needed a residential school, then her evidence would carry great weight. Unfortunately for her, this was to prove a political hot potato.

When I put my head around her door one day, she beckoned me to sit down for a moment. She told me that the education department of the Council had written to her about her report. They had asked her to explain her view that James needed a 24-hour communication programme. She had decided the letter was too political for her to deal with and so she had passed it to her boss. I didn't see the letter from the education department, but I did see a copy of the boss's reply and she wasn't budging:

'Having spoken to [James's speech and language therapist] I can clarify that James' needs are such that he needs to follow and be supported with his communication throughout his waking time over a 24 hour period in a consistent manner.

This could mean supporting him with his communication attempts in the same consistent manner if he wakes in the night.

A communication programme, developed and monitored by a speech and language therapist has been recommended in order that speech and language therapy targets can be integrated into his school and out of school life by carers and educational staff who have been trained in its delivery.

Please do not hesitate to contact me if further clarity is needed.'

I was elated when I read this. There was no fudging, it couldn't be clearer that the speech and language therapists were supporting me in getting a waking curriculum for James.

It was perhaps helpful that the speech therapists were employed by the NHS, not the Council, so they weren't at risk of losing their jobs if they failed to do what the Council wanted. However, even then it seemed that pressure had been brought to bear. In James's case the therapists withstood the pressure from the Council, but that isn't always so.

Two years later, I read of a case where a consultant who had diagnosed a child as autistic had later withdrawn her diagnosis under pressure from the education department of Essex County Council. The Council there didn't want to pay for the extra help involved in dealing with his special needs.[16] The father was a newsreader and so would have had an advantage in getting media exposure.

[16] *Laura Collins, The Mail on Sunday, 5 April 2009 page 15.*

I wondered if there were other parents who had had similar experiences, but who didn't have the connections to publicise their plight.

*

Soon after the speech and language therapist's report, the education department asked me for a meeting. They wanted to discuss my appeal against James's statement of special educational needs. I sat in a room with a couple of people and told them, carefully, why I wanted James to go to Dame Hannah Rogers School. They listened and made notes.

They told me that in July there would be a meeting of a multidisciplinary panel, which would include people from health and social care, to discuss James's needs. 'I'll put it in the diary', I said. They looked faintly embarrassed. 'You aren't allowed to attend', they said. I protested. 'You mean there is going to be an important meeting to discuss my son's future and I am not allowed to go?!' 'No' they said, and that was that.

Later, I obtained a copy of the minutes of that meeting. The panel thought that:

'...If domiciliary care is approved ... it may make a significant difference to providing support for Mrs Raca.'

They noted that an assessment with a view to providing this should have taken place earlier in the year (the one ordered by the independent reviewing officer in March after I had broken down), but this hadn't happened.

The panel went on to consider whether Tom (now aged nine) might be able to help me care for James, including changing his pad.

James is a large child for his age and can be very challenging. He requires regular changing due to his incontinence and two people are needed to safely carry out this and other tasks such as bathing, lifting and handling. It was agreed that it would not be appropriate to expect James's brother to assist with these tasks.'

I couldn't believe that they would even consider that Tom should be asked to help with the physical care of his incontinent brother! What century were we living in?

James's challenging behaviours were also recorded, with an open acknowledgement that he was not receiving all the therapy at school that he was entitled to because of lack of staff to deal with him ...

'[James's teacher] feels that a higher staff ratio would further benefit James as he can be very demanding. At present he has 2 people from Speech and Language to teach him PECS; this could be continued in class if there were more staff. ...

'[James's teacher] indicated that James does not always receive all he is entitled to, due to his behaviour and resistance in physiotherapy sessions'.

Finally, despite all of these admissions, the social worker asserted that even if I wanted them to, they wouldn't take James into care, as he wouldn't, in her opinion, meet the criteria for accommodation.

In July, I attended the LAC review which had been ordered as an emergency measure, three months after the last one. Social worker # 3 had disappeared and I met social worker # 4 for the first time.

The independent reviewing officer repeated the direction which had been made at the previous review, that the social worker should undertake an initial assessment of the family with a view to providing more support at home:

'Social Worker to discuss parents [sic] request for additional support and undertake an initial assessment...'Within one week of review.'

Social worker # 4 did arrange to meet us soon after the review, but I had to cancel as I had tribunal deadlines to meet. I called back twice to rearrange the meeting but didn't hear anything.

James then had an appointment with Dr R, the consultant who had taken over from Dr A, and who saw him for all his clinics at school. She knew about the tribunal, and in the manner I was used to from all the consultants and which I respected so highly, she pulled no punches: 'I have spoken to Dr A', she said, 'and she doesn't think you're going to win.' I didn't mind her saying this as I knew how hard it would be to win and was schooling myself to be prepared to lose. Even so, from such an authoritative source it was sobering. 'Why?' I asked. 'Well,' she said, 'They usually look at foster parents if the parents can't cope.'

I had never seriously thought the Council would consider foster parents, because James was so difficult to look after at home. It made no sense to me.

James needed to be in a residential school environment because only that could offer him the routines he needed in order to set him free from the prison of his own mind. When he was at school he was fulfilled. He could go out on trips and be meaningfully occupied.

If he carried on going to his day school, how would foster parents who barely knew him, be able to do what we who loved him deeply had failed to do – to find a way to help him live meaningfully outside school?

'No one would take him' I said. 'No one would be prepared to live with the broken nights and the poo fests.' 'I hope you're right' she said. 'Good luck.'

The schools broke up for the summer then, and we looked forward albeit uneasily, to two weeks in France without James. I didn't like leaving him for so long, but nothing would have made me give up those two weeks. For just a fortnight we could be a normal family, going on cliff walks, eating in restaurants without being attacked, lying on beaches and generally fooling around, without having to occupy, change, feed and wash James on a 24-hour basis. That summer was special, as Andrew and I celebrated our 15th wedding anniversary. We were both conscious of how close we had come to not having an anniversary to celebrate, and that made it particularly poignant.

In the autumn the expert social worker's report arrived. Because he was a solicitor as well as an experienced social worker, the report contained references to law.

For the first time I understood a little of the faceless 'court' that I had been dealing with, in the form of the social care department of the Council. I discovered that instead of a series of initial assessments by social workers, we should have had a core assessment, a much more detailed review of our family and its needs. Our expert wrote in his report:

'Analysis and Conclusions

72. I am particularly concerned that the Children's Services Department (as it now is) has failed to provide a Core Assessment of James Raca, despite not only the imperative of statutory guidance but the specific observations of at least one independent reviewing officer.

73. Failure to provide a Core Assessment has, albeit inadvertently, led to a situation where the local authority has, on several occasions, sent new social work practitioners into a complex situation, each without foreknowledge or understanding of the dynamics at play. In terms of contemporary social work practice, this is frankly inexcusable, though I hasten to add that it is essentially a managerial and systems failure, and not one attributable to the individual field workers...

75. All of the above suggests to me that the local authority is completely ill-equipped to provide, in holistic terms, the type and range of services which are now necessary to address the needs of James Raca and his family.'

He also said:

Parenting Capacity

'55...*I take the view that this is a family where the level of parenting is extremely high, and very distinctly moderated to ensure that James receives high levels of quality supervision and engagement...*

56. James's parents are wholly devoted to the care of their son. They have, at times, emotionally and physically succumbed to the unremitting pressures they are required to absorb, and they are able to address openly the fact that caring for James has been one critical component in their struggle to maintain equilibrium during very stressful times. Credit is due to them, in my opinion, because of their openness, and their honesty in stating the fact that 'care' for James is a massive, and sometimes especially onerous demand, not least because there are two other children who are entitled to parental nurture and care in equal measure within the family.'

The expert's comments about our parenting skills produced a big lump in my throat. Despite knowing that I had done my human best for all my children and my husband, I still felt that I had failed. That feeling hadn't been helped by some of the comments made by social workers in their notes, which I had seen in preparation for the tribunal. Now an 'independent expert' had assessed my parenting levels as extremely high. I shouldn't have needed that endorsement but I did. It was also to prove very helpful in the weeks to come, when my parenting skills were once again challenged by the Council.

Although my thoughts and energies were focused on the forthcoming tribunal hearing, I hadn't forgotten that officially we were supposed to be receiving more help at home. By mid-October I still hadn't heard from social worker # 4 so I wrote saying:

'I have a request for greatly increased respite and help which is outstanding from 20 March ... and I should like to discuss this.'

The social worker came to our house and announced that he was not familiar with our appeal to the tribunal and hadn't seen the evidence. Once again we were effectively faced with someone sitting down with a blank pad and a pen and saying 'So, tell me all about James.'

Wearily, I went once again through James's medical history, his life and the reason we were seeking a residential school for him. The social worker was very concerned about us and was a very kind man. He said that the Council's approach was to 'try to keep the family together'. They 'could look' at an extended package of support at home, and they could send people in to show me how to deal with James. I am afraid I actually laughed when he said this.

I suggested that I give him copies of all the evidence I had assembled for the tribunal and that he read it before we talked again. He thought that was a good idea until I appeared with two enormous files.

On his way out he mentioned that a core assessment had been done on the family. I stopped him in his tracks. The only contact with social care that anyone in the family had had since March was when I attended the LAC review at James's Birmingham school in July. It was now October. How could a core assessment have been done?

Social worker # 4 said he would send me a copy and left. He was as good as his word, and two days later a copy of a core assessment on the Raca family arrived in the post. It had been prepared by social worker # 2, apparently between June and October. Social worker # 4 had also signed it. It listed the agencies involved with the family and those who had been contacted.

There in black and white were the names of James's GP; his consultant Dr R; the occupational therapist; the nurse, head teacher and class teacher from James's Birmingham school; and the educational psychologist who had advised about James's challenging behaviours. Everyone in fact, except us! They had written what was supposed to be an in-depth report on our family, without contacting us at all.

I felt a deep sense of rage. My feelings weren't helped by some of the comments in the report such as:

'It is not clear the amount of emotional warmth James receives from his family...'

Almost as unbearable were the comments that suggested I had just given up on him, like a sink estate mother on crack cocaine:

'Ms. Raca is completely at a loss as to how to stimulate James in the home and finds it easier to simply leave him in front of the TV to watch videos. James obviously gets bored of this but Ms. Raca does not feel her home is designed to stimulate a child with autism...

'Ms. Raca is struggling to enforce any guidance and boundaries and finds the only way to get by at this stage is just to give in to James's demands.'

The report finally concluded that we needed more help at home:

'It is recommended that the best way of meeting James [sic] needs and to maintain him at home would be to provide additional support in the form of domiciliary care.'

By this stage we had been asking for more help at home for six months, but there was no sign of anything forthcoming.

*

In October I took James for the X-ray of his hips that had been suggested by the consultant at Dame Hannah Rogers School. I had written a letter to the hospital asking if they could do the X-ray in time for the tribunal, as the results might be helpful evidence. If the X-ray showed that James's hips had deteriorated (God forbid), there would be an arguable link between the lack of standing at school, where he was supposed to receive his therapy, and his physical condition.

That letter proved to be a big mistake.

On the morning of the appointment, James was being particularly difficult, and I was desperately trying to get him and Elizabeth ready, to load them into the little van which was adapted for the wheelchair. I was trying to drop Elizabeth off at school and get James to hospital on time. Tom had gone with a kind neighbour. On this day all my efforts failed. Elizabeth was still floating around in her snow white dress at 8.20am and the appointment was at 9am.

I didn't dare risk going to school and getting stuck in traffic. Elizabeth would have to come with us to hospital. I could really have done without coping with a four-year-old as well as James, but at least Elizabeth was totally enchanted that she got to miss school and wear her dressing-up clothes in public.

We got to the hospital to find that all of the disabled bays were taken. I had to park the little van on a double yellow line, put James's Blue Badge out and hope that we didn't get clamped.

I took James and Elizabeth into radiography reception and we waited. I hadn't given James any breakfast deliberately, so I could fill time in the waiting room by feeding him. I managed to make his marmalade sandwiches and grapes last about 20 minutes. Then we were called. 'Hooray' I thought. 'This is going to work after all.' I went up to the desk. The receptionist had a file open in front of her. I recognised my letter, asking for the appointment to be as soon as possible because of the tribunal.

'You want the X-ray as evidence for legal proceedings?' she said. 'Well', I said 'it depends what it shows, but maybe.' 'I am going to have to call someone', she said. 'Please take a seat.'

I sensed trouble and sat down apprehensively, keeping an eye on the desk. A little later, a woman in a suit appeared, her NHS identity card swinging on a ribbon around her neck. 'Are you Mrs Raca?' she enquired. I confirmed that I was. 'I am going to have to check the situation with this X-ray' she said. 'You may have to pay for it.' 'Why?' I asked. 'It's been ordered by his consultant.'

'I know', said the woman. 'But if you are obtaining evidence for the purpose of legal proceedings we have to charge you.'

James was beginning to get agitated and for once our emotions were synchronised. Elizabeth was spinning around, watching her skirt make a hemisphere like a jelly fish. 'Look, I have a daughter who should be at school and a severely disabled autistic son who will not cope with waiting here. He has an X-ray booked by his consultant because we need to check if his hips are coming out of their sockets. He should have had one done years ago. If the X-ray is helpful then I may use it in a legal case. I am not suing the hospital. This has nothing to do with the hospital.'

'I am sorry; I have to make enquiries' replied the woman, completely unmoved.

It wasn't so much the money she might charge, but the idea that I might have to be kept waiting with James and Elizabeth for hours, while this bureaucrat nit-picked about his X-ray. I lost my temper, something that doesn't happen very often, and I yelled at her. I told her to pick the bloody phone up and ring Dr R or Dr A.

'Please stop shouting at me' she said calmly and disappeared. She must have had NHS training in dealing with aggressive patients.

I sat down and wept. Then a woman who was sitting next to me, and who I had never met in my life, put her arm around me and drew my head onto her shoulder while I cried. 'Are you alone?' she asked. I nodded. I was alone that day. 'There, there' she soothed, in what sounded like a Scandinavian accent. 'There, there.'

Another golden nugget got stored in my heart, like the time the lady in Clinton Cards had given me a teddy with a lilac T-shirt, when James was having a tantrum.

The woman in the suit came back and told me briskly that it was all sorted out and James could go in for his X-ray now. I am afraid I was still not very polite to her.

James's hips were OK.

*

The tribunal was held in December 2007, just before Christmas. By the time it drew near I was so deep in preparations that I missed Elizabeth's first Christmas concert at school. I literally forgot. I went to pick her up and she was very brave at first, but gradually as she told me about being a shepherd, she burst into tears at the memory of searching for my face in the audience and not finding it. My friend Helen, whose daughter Alice was in the same class, had guessed what had happened and taken photos for me, but I knew that would never make it up to Elizabeth.

The intensity of that year took its toll. I had been conducting a legal case worth effectively £2 million. That was the reality of James's school fees, spread over 11 years from when he was eight to when he was 19 – the age allowed for disabled children to continue attending school. I was at the same time looking after three young children on broken sleep and mostly on my own, as Andrew was away in London all week. I would often fit an hour of work in before they rose and after I had returned from the school run; I would ignore absolutely everything else, including washing up, laundry, phone messages from friends, and just work.

The day would stop temporarily at 3pm, when I went on the school run again, and resume at 8pm when everyone was fed and bathed, and the two younger ones were tucked up. Then I would work until midnight or 1am.

I put on the 4 st that I had managed to lose after Elizabeth's birth and began to wheeze when I climbed up the stairs, as I had developed asthma. I was prescribed not only my first ever inhaler, but also a doubling of my dose of antidepressants.

Over the last few years, each time that life had felt vaguely balanced, I had stopped taking the tablets, only to find that I was waking up one morning at the bottom of a canyon again. I thought of it as a canyon because I had been to the Grand Canyon and seen how there was a wide river bed with another narrower one at the bottom of it, and another narrower one at the bottom of that.

I imagined that if you were at the bottom of the deepest river bed, you would climb up the sides and think you had reached the top of the canyon. Then you would realise that there was always yet another canyon to climb which you hadn't seen from where you were before. I thought depression was like that. When I was very low I didn't know how deep I had gone. When I was feeling a bit better, I thought I might be halfway up the canyon, when actually I had only gone up one river bed. Reaching the sunshine at the top was the objective, but being sure I had arrived was another goal which I hadn't achieved yet.

*

On the day, Andrew and I arrived at the place in Birmingham which had been booked for the tribunal hearing. We weren't in a formal courtroom, but in a meeting room in a hotel. I had obtained special dispensation for James not to be present, as I knew he would be very distressed and highly disruptive. It would have taken a judge's order to persuade me to collect him from school and bring him to that hotel.

Representing 'Team Raca' was our barrister, along with our expert physiotherapist, expert social worker, expert educational psychologist, me, Andrew and my mother. She was only an observer and wasn't allowed to speak, which must have been a great penance. Her presence, however, was crucial to us.

'Team Local Authority' comprised the head teacher of James's Birmingham school, the head of the school's physiotherapy department, a manager from social care, and another barrister.

The panel of judges was made up of three people, two were lay judges and the chair was a lawyer. It was the first time I had ever been in a court in the combined role of lawyer, witness and litigant and it felt very strange.

I wasn't technically representing our case but I would, in practice, support our barrister, as I had used to do in my previous life, by passing information to him and handing him documents which I thought might be helpful. I was glad that I had him by my side and that he was the expert who would be running the show. At that moment I was also relieved that I had chosen not to represent myself.

I was pleased that I had brought a big photo of James. We put it on the wall, so that in the middle of the politics we could all remember who we were talking about. It was the picture I had taken when he was put in the new style walker at Dame Hannah Rogers School and had gone marching down the corridor.

The hearing was listed for two days, which was unusual for this type of case, but then, as the expert educational psychologist said, 'Jane, these are the biggest bundles of evidence that I have ever seen!'

I don't remember everything about the hearing, only the ebb and flow and certain significant episodes. I learned from the local authority's barrister that the Council didn't include the services of an occupational therapist on the statements of children even as severely disabled as James, because they thought the physiotherapists could do the job.

With one policy decision, an entire profession - the occupational therapy profession - had been marginalised by the Council. The head of physiotherapy at James's Birmingham school said this decision was budget led.

Our independent expert physiotherapist was utterly indignant about the lack of time that James was spending at school in his standing frame. A report prepared by James's teachers for that year had said:

'He can walk/stand, supported by an adult, but constraints of staffing and time in school, mean this is only possible once a week generally, although he comes out of his wheelchair for at least a session daily.' [17]

'What is the point' she said, 'of saying that a child needs a standing frame, and then only putting him in it once a week?!'

There was a lot of argument over whether James was or wasn't making progress at his Birmingham school, but eventually I think it was our expert educational psychologist who turned things around.

She stood up and said we had to remember that for James education was about basic things. He was never going to take A levels or go to university. (At this point Andrew broke down and we paused the proceedings.) 'For James', she continued, 'education is going to be about more basic things such as learning to communicate.'

Our barrister, sensing we had a fair wind behind us, stood up and invited me to answer some questions.

'Jane, what would you like to see for James?' I took a deep breath: 'I want my son to learn to be able to walk and talk', I said. 'I want him to be somewhere where his therapy isn't just available on school days, but where people

[17] *When James came out of his wheelchair he would be crawling around, not standing or walking.*

are thinking about his posture and mobility at all times. I want him to be able to have a life where he can go out in the evenings and at weekends and isn't trapped inside the home, becoming more and more insular. He's disappearing inside himself', I said despairingly.

'The foods he's eating at home are becoming more and more restricted and there are fewer and fewer places that he will go. When he is at school he will eat anything and go anywhere.' I was talking so fast now that the barrister observed 'Jane, you need to slow down a bit, steam is coming off the judge's pen!'

When I had finished, Andrew stood up. At well over 6 ft tall he makes an imposing figure, especially when wearing a dark suit. I had finally managed to get out of leggings, but I was three sizes too big for my business suits and I had only just found the time to get a skirt and shirt for the hearing.

'When James was born', Andrew said slowly, 'I held my arms over his incubator. When he was diagnosed with cerebral palsy, I said to his consultant, "One day, he will stand up and be counted" and she said "I'm sure he will." Today is that day.' He paused. 'When I put James to bed at night we have a little routine. James likes me to walk him to the window, and he puts his hand on it and looks at me. And I say "Yes James, it's cold." Then he puts his hand on the radiator and looks at me again. And I say "Yes James, it's hot." He knows the difference between hot and cold. And he wants to hear me say it because he can't say it. He's very bright, but we can't give him what he needs at home. So we are showing our love for him by coming to this tribunal and asking for him to go to Dame Hannah Rogers School.' That was as far as he could manage before he broke down again, and so he sat down. Then, if I remember correctly, we adjourned for the day.

The barrister for the local authority was very clever and since he was trying to defeat our case I automatically disliked him.

There came a point where he kept repeating over and over that the way forward was for the Council to provide a package of domiciliary care which would help me to, among other things, 'Learn to communicate' with James. After I had heard this at least twice, I lost all sense of decorum and stood up in the middle of his submissions. 'Mr_ !' I said. 'Do you really think I don't know how to communicate with my own son?' There were a few moments of kerfuffle while Mr_ apologised for any misunderstanding.

The evidence about what James's Birmingham school could and couldn't do was dealt with, and there seemed to be no dispute about what Dame Hannah Rogers School could and couldn't deal with.

The Council presented its argument that James's educational needs were being met in Birmingham and that what we were looking for was just social care and support for us as parents. The manager from social care acknowledged that we had not had the support we might have anticipated and explained that the department had prioritised children in need of protection. These were children at risk of harm.[18] This had meant that children such as James ('children in need' simply by virtue of being disabled) tended to get put to the bottom of the pile. [19]

The manager said they had very recently restructured the department to separate out the two different sorts of case.

She announced that they could provide: 12 more nights at the Norman Laud Centre; one and a half hours of domiciliary care each weekday morning and evening; a parental support course through Barnado's (I never understood whether that was for us or James); and transport after school so that James could go to the after-school swimming and sports clubs. The manager said that a social worker would be allocated to make sure this all happened.

Our barrister asked me what I thought of this, did I think social care could deliver this package? I struggled to be polite and chose my words carefully. 'No' I said emphatically.

[18] *Children Act 1989 section 44(1).*
[19] *Children Act 1989 sections 17(1) and 17(10)(c).*

'You can't fix something that bad, that quickly.'

When it all ended, the chair explained that we weren't going to have the decision before Christmas, but she wished us a very merry holiday nevertheless. I wasn't disappointed as I knew we wouldn't get the decision that quickly anyway, but my mother seemed to read something into what the chair had said. 'I am sure she looked at me meaningfully' she said, 'when she wished me a merry Christmas.' 'Rubbish Mum!' I said heavily.

Outside the room, the social care manager came up to me. 'We need to put some extra support in place' she said. 'I'll give you a ring next week.'

Nothing happened.

We were numb all over the holiday, so numb that we weren't waiting in eager anticipation for the judgment, we were just, well, numb. Then it came, on a day of the week we weren't particularly looking out for it. It was a big heavy package. I opened it slowly and started to read through. My eyes swam. All I wanted to know was, had I got James into Dame Hannah Rogers School? I turned to the very back of the judgment, since the name of the school James should go to would be the last thing decided by the panel of judges.

It said 'Dame Hannah Rogers School.' I looked at Andrew. 'Do you think that means we have won?' We were so befuddled that neither of us dared take it in, but a little sparkler had been lit in our stomachs which gradually became brighter and brighter.

*

In 2007 Ofsted carried out its annual performance assessment of Birmingham City Council's children's services. Its report graded the services overall as good.

'The council has suitably responded to [the 2006 Joint Area Review] findings by implementing a strategy for children and young people with learning difficulties and/or disabilities. A new head of service has been established and the service is to be reconfigured. Some work has taken place to look at better integration of assessments and co-ordination of services.'

However the report also said:

'It is too early to judge the effectiveness of initiatives to improve services for children and young people with learning difficulties and/or disabilities. These services are being suitably restructured...' [20]

20 *Annual performance assessment of Birmingham City Council's children's services 2007. Ofsted, 26 November 2007.*

Chapter 11
A BETTER LIFE
2008

James's transfer to Dame Hannah Rogers School happened very fast. His Birmingham school gave him a good send-off, complete with a photo album of his time there. The guide who had been on his school bus every day for five years, told me in a confidential tone that there were some members of staff who thought I was getting rid of James but it was 'all right' because she knew it wasn't true. That pricked.

I went to say goodbye to those members of staff I had become fond of. I was relieved that they seemed to understand that I wasn't rejecting them or what they had done for James. The head of physiotherapy hugged me and said what had struck him during the tribunal hearing was our feelings for James. 'You just love him so much!' he said. The dinner lady asked for a photo of James to remember him by, and the head teacher asked me to keep in touch.

The person from the education department, with whom I had been dealing rather frostily during the tribunal process, called to discuss James's transfer. At the end of the call she hesitated: 'I've read so much about you,' she said. 'I feel as if I know you all really well!' I was too sore from the recent battle to take this as anything other than a further intrusion into my family's privacy. 'No Lady', I thought, 'you don't know us at all!'

The day arrived for James's first proper stay at Dame Hannah's and I went with him to Devon. The occasion didn't feel as dramatic as it could have done, since James was only going to be away for four weeks, then he would be coming home for half term. I was going to stay near him for the whole of the first week, in a holiday cottage I had rented. It would be only the second time that I had had a break from childcare since Tom was born, almost 11 years earlier, and I was really looking forward to it.

When we arrived, I was shown to James's bedroom. It had been newly decorated especially for him, with a bright blue carpet, a bright green beanbag and sea horses on the wall. The furniture was new, too. It was beautiful, just right for an eight-year-old boy and it broke my heart.

There was a picture window which came down below my knee level and which he might smash his way through. The sink was within easy kneeling reach, with lovely large-handled taps which James would turn on and off for hours and flood the room. There were mirrored tiles which he would bang his head against and break. The wardrobe was tall and freestanding, which he could pull over on top of himself. The staff had decorated the room for a little boy who couldn't move and didn't have autism, and the reality of what James was hit me anew.

I could hardly bring myself to tell them, but when I did he was instantly moved to another room of my choice. The second room was shabbier but had nothing dangerous in it, and with astonishing speed, a team of handymen had installed shelves at shoulder height which James couldn't reach, a plastic mirror, and a sink encased in a B&Q kitchen unit with a lockable lid. The room was painted to my specification (neutral as it would be more calming for James), and I had the luxury of going with the housekeeper to choose a new set of bed linen and curtains (neutral again). No effort was being spared to give James the right environment.

The handymen were a special feature of the school. The very nature of their job was to be instantly available to do bespoke work for the unique needs of the children. They could turn their hands to anything. In their spare time they built a hen house and a rabbit hutch in the school grounds and laid a wheelchair-friendly path, so the children could visit the animals. They sold the eggs laid by the hens to put into a fund for more equipment. As one of them told me, working at the school wasn't a job, it was a way of life.

I was comforted by the nurses' station just along the corridor from James, which was manned day and night. He would be checked every half an hour because of his epilepsy. Now if he seized in the early hours, someone would know about it.

I went with him into lessons. He now had his own support worker to help him. I watched him respond to the calm, very gentle teacher. Nothing happened suddenly and nothing was rushed. When it was his turn to say 'hello' using the sign of a raised thumb, everyone was going to wait as long as he needed. With the help of his support worker, he managed it.

On the walls of the corridor I noticed a list of 'Dos and Don'ts' for dealing with disabled people.

'Do look at me not my talker
Do give me a VERY long time to respond
Do talk to me at eye level
Do tell me when you want to move my chair – I am not a sack of potatoes
Don't lean on my device or my wheelchair without my permission
Don't switch off my device because I am being a pain or you disagree with me.'

James had a session with the speech and language therapist, where he had to choose an activity he wanted to do, by giving her a picture. He chose to listen to music, but she deliberately kept stopping the CD so he had to ask for it again.

He had a session on the trampoline where the physiotherapist made him bounce really high by jumping up and down next to him. He loved that. She made him ask for more bounces by stopping. He had to give her a card with a sign for 'more' before she would do it again. Then she did little bounces and asked him to choose between big bounces and little bounces using another card.

At lunchtime I found a place set for him with the right equipment and an eating plan stuck to his place mat, created by the occupational therapist. She had taken account of my concern that James was getting porky, and his puddings were restricted to apples and jelly. There was no concession to his obsession with ham sandwiches and crisps. He would have whatever was cooked.

Many of the more vulnerable children had food tailor made for them. Some had cooked food which had been liquidised. For some even that was too much and they were fed via gastrostomy tubes which went straight into their stomachs. For them lunch was a special milkshake which by-passed their mouths completely. The staff would still say, 'ummmmmm lunch now', as if they were going to share a banquet.

In the evenings I went back to my holiday cottage on the Moors, felt the wind blowing through my hair and was at peace. I read, went for walks and enjoyed the silence in my head.

The end of the week came and it was time to say goodbye to James until he came home for half term three weeks later. I could cope with leaving him because I could see that already he was opening up to the staff at Dame Hannah's like a sunflower. However, I still drove away from the school feeling a confused mix of sadness, relief and exhaustion.

Arriving home was also strange. The absence of James was a tangible thing because when he was there he was such a dominating presence, with his all-consuming needs. Over the next few days, my emotions fluctuated violently between euphoria that I could finally rely on an uninterrupted night's sleep and awe at the enormity of the change I had wrought. I wandered into his empty bedroom, with all the disabled equipment in it, and was overcome with grief at the absence of one of my children.

I slept a great deal and it was around this time that Tom, now aged ten, wrote a poem at school which was more poignant than he could possibly have imagined.

'My Mum is very nice.
I don't think she has head lice
But she often scratches her head
And spends lots of time in bed.'

It was to be the beginning of a new dynamic for the four members of the family who were left. At first there was a large James-shaped hole, but not because everyone missed him. I don't think the other children did miss him. From their perspective he had often been violent, aggressive and selfish towards them.

As for Andrew and I, James had just taken up so much of our time and energy that we weren't sure what to do with all the free time we now felt we had. In reality, we had been so used to spending all our waking hours running between practical tasks that to have even half an hour to read a newspaper seemed the highest form of luxury. In turn, the other children had become so used to having very little of us that they continued in their self-sufficient way for a while. Slowly though, the James-shaped hole was to become smaller and the relationship the rest of us had with each other changed and reformed. It was to take us three years before we all, including James, settled down into this new life. By then it had begun to feel normal and to have a rhythm of its own, which we all understood.

James had been given a houseparent at the school, and she wrote home to us on a weekly basis. We read her letters with disbelief and exultation at the extent of the activities that James was now doing.

James has enjoyed lots of different activities this week including maple dancing… parachute and ball games in the garden, a day at Paignton zoo, a boat show on Plymouth Hoe, walks in the park and a music and movement night.' [21]

A music and movement night! He wouldn't have done that at home. He would have been trapped in front of *Teletubbies*.

The Easter holidays began and since the Birmingham schools broke up a week earlier than Dame Hannah's, we decided to rent a holiday cottage for a few days so we could go and see James in his new environment. We didn't want him to feel that his life was sharply divided between Birmingham where he saw us, and Devon where he didn't. We went to Dame Hannah's and sat in his bedroom all watching *Postman Pat* together. We swam in the hydrotherapy pool at school as a family. It was as big as a small swimming pool and had some special features. James could touch switches at the side of the pool to make disco lights and music. The pool was so hot we almost fainted. It had to be that way, so that the more vulnerable children didn't become very cold while their muscles were being stretched with exercises in the warm water. Then James came home again.

I noticed that the staff had taught him a sign for 'please', which he was also using as 'yes'. He simply tapped the wrist of his left hand with his right hand. It made a massive difference to his ability to tell us what he wanted. Now we could say, 'James, would you like some toast?' And he could say 'yes'. If he didn't say 'yes' it meant 'no', so now he could say 'yes' and 'no'.

He used this new sign when he had a seizure. He obviously knew he was about to be ill and started tapping his wrist over and over. I said 'What is it James?' Then I saw what the problem was and held him while he had the fit. It wasn't the clearest use of 'yes' and 'no', but it was the way he knew he could get our attention.

---

[21] *All extracts from letters from James's carers are quoted as written.* **181**

*

As the year progressed, I had heard nothing more from the social care department since the tribunal, and I was in a no-man's-land as far as respite was concerned. James was at Dame Hannah's for three terms, but the holidays were anyone's guess.

I knew I ought to find out what the position was, but I was so weary of the Council and also wary, that I couldn't bring myself to get in touch and clarify the situation. Eventually though I had to, as the holidays were looming and I couldn't go back to having James at home with no help. He was now used to one-to-one supervision, all the time, and would be even more difficult to handle at home if he didn't have it.

Social worker # 4 had disappeared, and we had yet another social worker, # 5. She came to the house and I explained to her all about the tribunal. I told her that James had been promised domiciliary care by the social care manager who had been there, but I hadn't heard anything. She told me that the manager who had been at the tribunal was her boss and was leaving a few days later, so I had better act quickly. I was keen that it was that manager in particular who dealt with the respite, as she had heard all the evidence at the tribunal about James's extensive needs.

I wrote a three-page letter summarising the evidence from the tribunal and explaining that I needed clarification soon. The respite provision both at Norman Laud and at Dame Hannah's was getting booked up for the summer. I rang twice afterwards to try to catch her before she left. Nothing happened.

A few weeks later I rang the disabled children's team to see if I could find out what was going on. Someone went to look at the file and told me that James's respite allowance of 60 nights had been cancelled, since he now had the placement at Dame Hannah Rogers School. A feeling of disbelief swept over me. Despite the tribunal evidence having proved that he needed one-to-one or even two-to-one care all the time, the Council was planning to leave him unsupported for 14 weeks of school holiday per year! We wouldn't be able to go anywhere with the other children, we would all be trapped in the house again.

My dismay was deeper for having won the tribunal. Naively, I had assumed that having proved the extent of James's needs in a legal forum – having had them recorded in black and white in a judgment – that that would be the end of all the fighting. One of the first lessons I had been taught at law school in the 1980s was 'never assume'. It was to haunt me painfully for the next three years.

After my phone call, social worker # 5 came to visit me again. This time she was accompanied by her new manager, as the one who had been at the tribunal had now left. This manager looked quite fierce.

She said that if we wanted James to spend more than 38 weeks (three terms) away from home, then there was a procedure to follow to protect his interests. The Council needed to ensure that he was not unnecessarily being deprived of his family and his home. He would have to become a 'looked after child' (nothing new there) and the social worker would have to make a request to a specialist panel for funding for the holidays. The panel was necessary because the funding for the placement would be split between education, social care and health. The social worker would have to show how the input James received was split between those three departments, so the panel could apportion the budget.

I wondered how on earth I could break down what happened to James at Dame Hannah's into health, education and social care. Everything was multidisciplinary, so that during lunchtime he might eat, use his hand signs and picture communication and also wear his leg gaiters.

Fortunately that was not my job, the Fierce Manager said. The school would provide information about that. My primary input would be to show what level of contact James would have with his family for such extended periods away. I should quote the level of contact we had already had. I could even supply petrol receipts and expenses to back it up.

Petrol receipts to prove I loved my son! After everything that had been said at tribunal! The ignominy of it left me reeling again. My face must have betrayed how I felt, as the Fierce Manager said perhaps I didn't need petrol receipts. But I wasn't going to take any chances. If I might need petrol receipts, they would get petrol receipts.

I wasn't going to be allowed to attend the panel meeting that would decide on the respite allowance, just as I hadn't been able to attend the one that took place the previous year, where they had considered whether Tom, aged nine, could help me with James's care.

Before she left, the Fierce Manager expressed an interest in James's autism and the fact that he only ate a limited diet at home. She said she was a holistic therapist and was interested in the use of diet to manage conditions like his. She suggested that I try celery, fennel, balsamic vinegar and Chinese beans. I imagined what James would do if I presented him with a plate of these things. A vision of them being thrown all over the Fierce Manager came into my head and I had to stifle a giggle.

Later that month I heard in the news of the death of a little girl called Khyra Ishaq. She had starved to death in her own home, even though social workers in Birmingham had been alerted and had visited the house. I thought of the comments that the social care manager had made at James's tribunal, that 'children in need of protection' were dealt with by the same social workers as 'children in need' just because they were disabled. If the service failed children who needed protection, no wonder that children who were a lower priority, such as James, had to battle for any provision at all.

We got another letter from James's houseparent at Dame Hannah's. James had gone to an evening show, ridden his bicycle around and was learning to make a sandwich.

'He went to see Bob the builder live on stage at the pavilions last night– which he just loved! All the characters trucks and diggers were life size. James watched in amazement.'

'He bought a blue bob the builder cup out of his pocket money which he loves drinking out of. He's had to get the hang of making sure all his drink is gone before he can turn it around and look at all the pictures very closely as he does...'

'Friday brings with it cooking day. He is beginning to show the first signs of understanding the sequencing needed in making the sandwich rather than just seeing it all as food which needs to be eaten immediately! Saying that though, eating the food is still a highly motivating factor of this session!'

*

In June I turned up for a LAC review, to find that the venue had been rearranged without anyone telling me. Social worker # 5, and the independent reviewing officer were in Devon, and I was in Birmingham. It was the beginning of a series of episodes where the meetings seemed to be organised for the convenience of the officials and I was forgotten.

Now that James was at school in Devon it transpired that his LAC reviews had to be held there. Consequently, that made a big impact on the diary of the Birmingham Council staff who had to travel to attend. It also meant that it was more difficult for me, as I had to arrange childcare for Tom and Elizabeth overnight. I dared not miss the reviews. However, if a meeting in Devon was rearranged at short notice, or worse, without anyone telling me, it was very stressful.

By the beginning of July, I had put together a report for social worker # 5 as the Fierce Manager had asked. I had gone further than the petrol receipts showing we visited

James. I had also re-copied evidence from the tribunal, as to why James needed extra support when he was at home, and why he needed to be at Dame Hannah's for most of the year. It was ludicrous that I felt obliged to do this after all that we had already proved at the tribunal, but if that was what it took, then that is what I would do. It seemed to me that the Council was determined to reinvent the wheel, so I was going to give the social worker all the ammunition I could. She had told me that she would use the evidence to present our case to one specialist children's panel, which would then take the matter to a second specialist panel.

Two weeks later she rang me very pleased to say that the First Panel had recommended a total 48-week placement at Dame Hannah's. That was ten weeks of respite for the school holidays, on top of the three terms (38 weeks) which the tribunal had ordered.

The First Panel wanted her to seek our views. I said we were very happy with that. She said the matter would go to the Second Panel the following week, but she wouldn't be allowed to attend.

I waited anxiously by the phone on the day of the Second Panel meeting, to hear the outcome. The summer holidays loomed and I had no provision for help with James – either respite at Dame Hannah's or funding for a carer at home.

No one rang.

I rang the disabled children's team, only to be told that social worker # 5 was off sick. I wrote in despair to the Fierce Manager and got a message back that no decision had been made by the First Panel. I didn't understand that.

Finally, in September, social worker # 5 returned to work and rang me to tell me the outcome of the Second Panel meeting that had been held in July. It wasn't what I wanted to hear. The Second Panel had said the issue was not their responsibility to consider!

Our application was now floating in some no-man's-land between the two Panels.

The social worker, who had been so triumphant at convincing the First Panel of our case, was clearly disturbed by this. She gave me a copy of an email she had been sent by the Council at the beginning of the whole process. It confirmed what she said she had been told, that she would attend the meeting of the First Panel and they would take the matter to the Second Panel.

I later got hold of the minutes of the meetings of the two Panels. The matter had gone right round in a circle, starting with social care, then going to the First Panel, then the Second Panel, and then being referred back to social care with no resolution.

It was to take me another two and a half years to get that resolution.

The failure of the system to come up with an answer to our request for support in the holidays meant that despite everyone agreeing that James needed one-to-one, sometimes two-to-one, care all day long, we had no respite for the school holidays. We also had no domiciliary care for when he was home. In this year James came home with no financial provision for the whole summer.

We were in a worse position in some ways than when he had been at his Birmingham school. Then we had used our respite allowance so that Andrew, Tom, Elizabeth and I could go away as a family, for a break which James would have found intolerable.

Now we had James at home for all six weeks of the school summer holidays.

It was unthinkable to manage alone, so we asked James's houseparent from Dame Hannah's, Lucy, to come and live with us, *au pair* style, to help. We were lucky enough to have savings to pay her and she, in turn, was saving to go travelling round the world for a year. She needed the money, she loved James and so she agreed.

The holiday started with us all going to Devon to spend a few days with James when he broke up and to take him to the beach. The staff didn't normally take the children out of their wheelchairs onto the beach, as most were too medically vulnerable, with gastrostomy tubes or oxygen tanks. Also, accessing the beach was a challenge in a heavy wheelchair, which wasn't designed to travel across sand. However, we found a beach with a slipway and managed to get James into the sea.

He knelt in the waves at the edge like King Canute and bounced for joy. Wave after wave broke over him, he was knocked over by the surf, but his face shone with exhilaration at the feel of the wet sand, the echoing 'ark ark' of the sea gulls and the white foam swirling around him.

As we made our way back, I made the mistake of talking in front of James about the fact that Lucy would be leaving at the end of the summer to go travelling. Andrew had warned me not to do this, but I had forgotten to take care. After a moment James started to cry in a terrible way, with real tears and sobs. I realised that he had understood what I had been talking about and didn't want Lucy to go. I felt awful.

When we got back home to Birmingham, Lucy was amazed at how differently James behaved there compared with at school. She became determined to get him to eat cooked food with a spoon like he did at Dame Hannah's and tucked them both away in the utility room on their own while she tried to persuade him to do it. After a number of days she was successful, but it took longer to get him to come and share a meal with us in the kitchen.

She had never seen James have a real tantrum, but one day in Birmingham she tried to take him to the cinema, not realising that it didn't have disabled access. James went berserk and pulled one of her earrings out, ripping her ear lobe. She was a brave, resilient girl, but she was upset and shocked by his aggression.

Having Lucy with us that summer really saved us. She

sat and watched *Teletubbies* with James for hours on end; she went with him into town on the bus to wander round the shops; she also helped me take him swimming in our local pool.

Our first outing to the swimming pool was eventful. We hadn't taken him before, as he had always swum in the pool at his day school when he lived in Birmingham. On this occasion we were therefore unprepared for James's interest in his fellow public swimmers.

While Lucy swam a few lengths to get warm, I stayed with James, who was happily paddling in his armbands in the big pool. There was no one within several feet of him, so I decided I could swim widths nearby. I had just reached the side of the pool and turned round, when I saw an elderly bald man doing a slow front crawl, going right in front of James. To my utter horror, James grabbed the man by the neck in a trice and started to chew his ear! I swam as quickly as I could towards them, but nothing would have been fast enough. I felt as if I were in one of those nightmares where you are trying to run away from a monstrous beast but your feet are stuck in the mud. The man's eyes bulged out of his head in shock and fright, while James grinned and chewed. 'No James!' I cried, and he immediately let go. He was usually quite good like that. The man swam off, traumatised.

On subsequent visits to the pool, we didn't leave James unattended for a second. He developed a particular fondness for toddlers, especially if they were crying, which he thought was very funny.

Eventually the long summer was over, Lucy went travelling and James went back to Devon. I had been immersed in the intensity of his presence just as it used to be before the tribunal. Even with Lucy's help, the demands had been unbearable and James had suffered through not having enough things he could do and from the lack of physiotherapy. We had also not used PECS all summer and school noticed a regression.

Once term had started we began to get letters from James's houseparent at Dame Hannah's again. I had sent some photos of the family back with James when he went home at the end of the summer and these proved a great hit.

James loves his new photos, especially the one with his Mummy, himself, Tom and Elizabeth. The first thing James does in the morning when I go into his room is showing me the photos of you all. Then I have to ask him 'Where is your Mummy, or where is your Daddy?' and he shows the right photos. This is our morning game. Sometimes I ask him about his Polish Babcia and he looks at me and then shows the window which of course means she is not here. He is so clever!'

I started to write regularly to James and to put a photo of the family on my letters. These became important to all of us. The staff laminated them and kept them in a folder for James to look at.

James really enjoys your letters and his chocolate buttons, he was so good with the last letter he was very gently with it after I had read it to him he held it and looked at the pictures of you all for quiet a while after lunch, James still holding his letter went to his room showing nicely other members of staff his letter on the way.'

His bedroom at school was very bare, deliberately so because it helped keep him calm. However, I thought it would be nice to get him a few blown-up pictures of the family to go on his walls, so I went online and ordered three. Unfortunately I didn't research sizes first and ordered them in A1 size, thinking it was a quarter of the size of an A4 piece of paper. (In fact A1 is eight times the size of an A4 piece of paper.) When the posters arrived and I unfurled them from their cardboard tube, a giant picture of my head emerged, the size of a dinner plate. James now had a larger than life-sized Mummy grinning down at him, like a deity, as he slept.

*

With the children back at school I could once again tackle the piles of paper on the dining room floor. I wrote to our local councillor and our MP, asking if they could help resolve the impasse about respite and help for James in the holidays. They both wrote to the Council's social care department and less than a month later I got a response from a manager at the disabled children's team. He apologised for the confusion and said that he would reinstate the 60 nights of respite James had used to spend at the Norman Laud Centre, and that he could take it at Dame Hannah's. When added to the 38 weeks we had been awarded at the tribunal, it made a rather strange package of 46 weeks and 4 days in total, but was a significant improvement. The manager also said he would fund a carer to be with James for ten hours per day when he was at home.

My shoulders sagged with the relief of knowing that we didn't have to face every school holiday with James at home. At the same time I had a lump in my throat at the black and white reality of what I had done. My son was only going to come home for a few weeks each year. He was really going to be living elsewhere and he was only nine.

The letter didn't say when the new package would start, but it all sounded as if it was being sorted out and I looked forward to having help in time for the Christmas holidays. The letter was not in time for us to get help for the October half term though, so once again we were thrown back to pre-tribunal times. By the end of that week, having looked after all three children on my own night and day, I was returned to the zombified state of 2007. Poor Tom and Elizabeth had spent the entire time holed up watching TV in a separate room to James. The one consoling factor was that, demonstrating the influence of Dame Hannah's, James had eaten cornflakes and milk with a spoon for the first time.

The letters from the school continued to arrive, giving voice to James's personality in the same way as the card which had been made by the staff at his Birmingham school, when I had been in hospital pregnant with Elizabeth.

I loved reading what he had been doing and how he amused everybody with his antics. I also had a deep, quiet joy in knowing how full his life was now that he was no longer imprisoned in a playroom, with his head inside an infant television programme.

'We had a Halloween party at school this week... Fed and giggling, James could watch a fireworks show in the school garden. I thought he would be afraid. But I was so wrong. He loved that! He kept looking at fireworks and when the sky got black again he reached for my hand and then pointed at the dark sky and then looked at me again and it was so clear he asked me for more.

So the only thing I could do was just show him my empty hands and say 'I've got nothing'. That makes him laugh. And that's our new game. It's a good calmer as well and it works every time.'

I knew that if I had tried to take James to a fireworks display in Birmingham he would have had a serious tantrum.

In November it was once again time for James's LAC review. The social worker told me that the Council wasn't happy with the 46-week and 4-day placement promised by the manager, because it should technically be 48 weeks. She was going to have to go back to the First Panel again to try to get the placement increased. In the short term, the manager was going to fund a carer to come home with James for Christmas, on a one-off basis.

The people at the Council who crunched numbers were

also not happy with the unusual length placement and refused to pay the school's first invoice until I faxed them the manager's letter.

In the meantime, the school and I decided to assume that James's 46-week and 4-day placement would begin by Christmas. This mattered, since at that time, if James's placement was for more than 42 weeks, by law he had to be in a children's home. He would move from the boarding wing of the school to a beautiful purpose-built bungalow in the grounds.

The staff started a careful process of taking him over there and letting him choose his own room so that he was comfortable about what was, for him, a massive change.

When I went to visit him in December, the night staff told me how he had crawled out of bed and had cunningly crept around the back of the nurses' station so that they didn't see him entering the lounge. They had found him happily watching *Postman Pat* at 3am.

We received a final letter from his houseparent before he broke up for Christmas.

'Wednesday was a lovely day. After circle time James enjoyed a lovely trip out to the Donkey Sanctuary. He had a ride on the donkey-cart which was all decorated up. The cart took him to see Father Christmas. James was able to tell Father Christmas (with his big mac [talker]) that he had been a good boy this year. Father Christmas congratulated him and gave James a present!'

James arrived home and for the first time we had funding from the Council for the carer who came with him. As with having Lucy in the summer, it helped to have another pair of hands, but we still found his visit almost intolerable.

It was a bad time of year for him to be home, as going out was more difficult in the dark and cold, so we were all stuck inside even more than usual. Perhaps more significantly, I was also trying to have a 'proper' family Christmas. After the short cuts I had taken to survive his years at home, like buying a lot of frozen pizza, I was now trying to give the other children a taste of the sort of Christmases I had enjoyed as a child. I wanted to make a Christmas cake and actually put up the Christmas cards. The reality was that we were getting used to not having James around for a lot of the time – the peace and extra time had stopped being novel and simply felt normal. So while it was wonderful to see James, I did also feel as if I were being plunged back into the hell of pre-tribunal times.

*

In December 2008 Ofsted prepared its annual report into Birmingham City Council children's services. The Report found that overall, these services were performed adequately. However, it identified important weaknesses and areas for development in relation to vulnerable groups.

'Action to deliver ambitions, improve services and remedy the areas for development identified in the 2007 APA [Area Performance Assessment] letter has been inconsistent. As a result, performance has deteriorated in some outcome areas, particularly for vulnerable groups...
    ' *Serious shortages in the social care workforce, together with a sharp drop in the percentage of residential case workers with NVQ Level 3 in health and social care, impacts negatively on the council's capacity to fully deliver social care services efficiently and effectively.*' [22]

[22] *Annual performance assessment of services for children and young people in Birmingham City Council 2008. Ofsted, 17 December 2008.*

Chapter 12
TIME TO CLEAR THE WRECKAGE
2009

In the New Year of 2009, social worker # 5 rang me to talk about the meeting of the First Panel she had just attended, to have another go at getting the 48-week placement at Dame Hannah's for James. She was sorry to say that their decision had been postponed. The First Panel wanted a report from the education department before making a decision about joint departmental funding.

In the February half term James had an appointment at the wheelchair clinic in Birmingham. He had outgrown his wheelchair and had to be specially measured for a new one. Like the wheelchair he had been in when he fell off the roundabout, it would need to have straps to keep his feet from sticking straight ahead of him, a large belt around his waist, and a five-point harness on his chest. It would be measured to fit his legs and torso and would be very heavy, with a tall headrest and stabilisers at the back for when he rocked. Although he was now registered with the health service in Plymouth, Dame Hannah's told me that Plymouth would not accept responsibility for his wheelchair, so I had to get it from Birmingham.

When James had been at his Birmingham school, the wheelchair clinic had been held there. Now that he had left that school he had to go to a clinic at a hospital. We hadn't been there before. I knew that taking James in the car to a strange place would be likely to trigger a tantrum, so I planned the trip with military precision. I filled the car up with petrol the day before so we didn't have to stop at a garage with James. I did a test run to see how long the journey took so we could leave in sufficient time to keep the appointment, but were not so early that we would have to wait around. That would only make James anxious. I packed chocolate buttons and a photo of me. It was strange, but photos of me could sometimes calm him more than the real me, and he could bite the photo with impunity. Finally, I took a portable DVD player with *Teletubbies* on, so he could be kept in his own green and pleasant land of Laa-Laa and Po.

We had a rocky start as he didn't want to get in the car, so he attacked me and the carer. We produced calming aid number one, the photo of me, which worked. We got him in, clutching the photo, and strapped him up. I started the car, drove forward and then paused briefly as I exited the drive, to check I wasn't running anyone over. This temporary stop was enough to send James into hysterics, so out came the DVD with *Teletubbies* on. As we drove to the wheelchair clinic, he was quieter, but there was still an underlying tension in the car, a sense of pent-up menace. When we arrived and parked, I gave James my final offering, the chocolate buttons, to help him cope with the car having stopped.

He ate them in seconds and then, as I leant across him to undo his seatbelt, talking softly and kissing him, he sank his jaws into my chin like a terrier and clawed my face. I knew he was very frightened and anxious, which is why he was doing it, and I wasn't angry with him. I was, though, shocked and upset at the violence of his attack.

The carer and I managed to grapple him into his chair, but he was throwing himself about wildly as we went into reception and neither of us dared get anywhere near to him. The staff took pity on us and we were shown straight through, but I was crying and couldn't speak for the first ten minutes.

I left to go to the ladies toilet to check my bleeding chin, while the carer, who was also shocked but unhurt, spoke to the technicians. Fortunately, James was calmed by being in a small room with them. They were polite and comfortable with him, describing him as their client and talking to him rather than about him. Eventually my sobs were all spent and they said that next time he was assessed for a new wheelchair they would come to the house.

I was filled with gratitude and made a mental note to ask for a home appointment for everything for James from now on.

My gratitude partly evaporated though, when I had to fill in some forms at the end of the appointment and wrote down James's GP's address in Devon. 'Oh,' they said, 'Why is his GP in Devon?' I told them about the school and they shook their heads sorrowfully. 'We can't treat him any more,' they said. 'We'll do this chair but next time he will have to be seen by his local service. Patients here have to be registered with a Birmingham GP.'

I thought of what Dame Hannah's had said, that Plymouth didn't pay for the wheelchairs of Birmingham children. I wondered what would happen in two years' time when James would need a new wheelchair and Birmingham wouldn't provide it either. The cold dull feeling came over me. I had always stuck to the principle of being scrupulously honest and not exploiting James's disability in order to get help or sympathy. Perhaps I should abandon that now and become a renegade. I could tell a lie and register him with a GP in both areas just before the next wheelchair assessment. That way I might get the chair before anyone found out. I might even get two chairs! I was appalled at where all this struggling was taking me.

The letters from James's houseparent continued to arrive and to provide an antidote to the heartache. I read of how he went wheelchair line dancing and to a masked ball, where he made the mask. He was learning to recognise the shape of a word so he could choose a card with the name of the object he wanted, rather than a picture, to ask for it. He had also been to watch a football match.

'On Saturday James enjoyed a trip out. We had a picnic at Central Park before we went into watch the football. James was happy and smiley and enjoyed the music and the mascot that goes to greet the children and throws sweets for everyone to catch. James really enjoys this you can tell by the look on his face. During half time James enjoyed listening to the bag pipes that were being played he loved it and was dancing away in his chair I wasn't sure James would enjoy the noise but he loved it and was signing for 'more' when they had finished.'

He had a new houseparent who wrote funny letters. She told us how she had taken him into Boots the chemist and let him smell the hand creams for a sensory experience. Then she had started to massage some into his arm, only to find it was exfoliating scrub! She had quickly left the store.

*

In March, my friend Joanna and I finally got to the pub, nearly three years after she had first suggested it. It was the beginning of Lent and I had resolved to give up alcohol. I knew Joanna always did. As evening approached I thought of sitting in the pub all evening nursing tonic water. Joanna came round at 7pm and we started walking up the road. 'It's St Joseph's Day', she said. 'Who's he?' I asked naively, Bible studies not having been a significant feature of my childhood. 'You know', she said. 'Jesus' father!' 'Oh, I didn't know he was a saint', I said. 'Yes' she replied, 'he's my favourite saint. Little known and much underappreciated. I think we should celebrate him.' 'What a good idea' I said. Several hours and many glasses of wine later, Joanna and I waltzed into my house giggling. Joanna had persuaded me that saints' days didn't count for Lent.

James came home again at Easter and this time he was better behaved than on the previous visit. We stuck carefully to going only to very familiar places. He tolerated walking around the reservoir as long as we fed him frequently. We tried to wean him off this, but had to concede defeat when he began eating the bushes near to the path. He had a crafty tactic: he would point at a particular shrub and Lauren (the carer) or I would obligingly push him nearer for a good feel, a bit of sensory experience. Then he would stuff his mouth full of leaves and munch. He was indiscriminate, once even grabbing a bunch of nettles. Lauren said that they had nettle-eating competitions in Devon and she would enter him next time, as she was sure he stood a good chance.

As well as feeling bushes, he liked to stroke the dogs that frequently passed us. This made us very tense as 'stroking' wasn't quite what he had in mind. The owners would see his interest in their beloved pet and be very keen to allow the little disabled boy a pat. When Lauren and I tried to keep James away they would say 'It's alright, he won't bite!' What they didn't know was, we weren't afraid for James, we were afraid for the dog!

In April I had a phone call from another social worker. There was a LAC review coming up in May. Social worker # 5 had left and the new social worker, # 6 would be attending.

I explained that we still had no money to cover the summer holidays which were rapidly approaching, despite a letter from the manager in February, saying that direct payments for a carer at home had been agreed. I also had no information as to what had happened about getting approval from the First Panel or the Second Panel for the 48-week placement at Dame Hannah's.

Social worker # 6 said he would try to get up to speed in time for the LAC review. I thought it unlikely he would be able to get on top of James's case by then. I wrote to the manager asking what was going on. I told him of my despair at never knowing whether or when funding was going to be forthcoming for a particular holiday, making booking the carers or family holidays away without James very difficult.

The day of the LAC review arrived. I noticed it was now called a 'child in care' (CIC) review. I didn't think of James as a child in care. I asked the independent reviewing officer what he thought about the situation with James's package. Did these Panels really need to agree his placement? It seemed to be a very difficult process.

The independent reviewing officer said that indeed James's overall placement did need to be agreed by the Second Panel. He explained that while the 38-week term-time placement was funded jointly by health, social care and education, the respite provision for the holidays was funded solely by social care. The manager who had promised to fund it might leave and his successor might not honour the agreement.

Now I understood! I thought of what would happen if social care decided to cut the respite again, as they had first done when we won the tribunal. I imagined having James home for all the holidays, which made up 14 weeks of the year. I thought of how he might suffer if his placement was only 38 weeks, because he might have to move from the children's home, back to the boarding wing of the school. He hated change. The social work assistant told me he would take the matter to whichever was the appropriate Panel.

By mid-June nothing had happened. I wrote again to my councillor and MP. All three of us wrote to the manager who finally replied three days before James broke up for the summer. He said he would fund a carer for the summer holiday. In relation to the 48-week placement at Dame Hannah's, he apologised for the delay and said he would take personal responsibility to ensure progress was now made.

'I had asked that the Team Manager to [sic] follow up the issues raised regarding the securing Tripartite funding for James's placement at Dame Hannah Rogers for 48 weeks. Unfortunately the Team Manager left the Directorate and this matter had not been progressed in the manner that I had

requested. I accept that this is not acceptable and have taken personal responsibility to ensure progress is now made ...

'Please accept my apology for any inconvenience caused by the delay in progressing this matter. I am aware of the pressures and strain involved in caring for a child with profound and complex disabilities and I am sorry for any additional stress caused by the delay in resolving this matter.'

In normal circumstances I would have been pleased and relieved to get this letter, and full of good feelings. However, I was now becoming deeply cynical.

I had become used to experiencing chaos from the Council and to things not happening. Now I was getting used to promises being made and not kept. At least I could get through the next few weeks, but I wondered what would happen after that.

*

In the summer I went to visit James. I had begun to take him swimming in the leisure centre near to Dame Hannah's. The pool there was bigger and cooler than the tropically heated hydrotherapy pool at the school, where he had his stretches with the physiotherapist. He didn't go to the leisure centre as part of his life at school, as many of the children were too vulnerable to contemplate taking to a public pool, with its chlorine and germs. A visit just for him alone would require two carers and he was only funded for one. So I liked to give him a treat when I visited, something special that he only did when Mummy came. I had to be careful not to spend too much time talking to the carer though, as James would get jealous and hit me lightly to tell me to talk to him instead.

When we arrived on this occasion we found that half of the pool was roped off for an over-60s session. The pool was kidney shaped, which looked stylish but made swimming lengths rather tricky. With half of it roped off, the people hoping to do serious exercise would be cramped.

The carer and I were staying close to James (we didn't want a repeat of the ear-chewing incident). A mother had left her tiny child with its grandma in the baby pool, while she frantically tried to snatch a few minutes of fast swimming. As she approached the natural turning point, at the longest part of the kidney, she found James having a splash. She surfaced for a moment from her front crawl and looked at me. 'I am sorry', I said. 'Are we in your way?' 'Yes' she said, unsmiling. I decided then and there that I wasn't going to move and neither was James. This woman would have many years ahead of her when her child could walk and swim and she could do as many lengths as she liked. She would have to wait until then.

*

In the autumn I received a letter from Plymouth NHS telling me of an appointment that James had with his orthopaedic consultant.

I realised that I couldn't go. I had no cover for Tom and Elizabeth that week. The tone of the letter didn't suggest that I could ring up and rearrange the appointment: it was formal, even faintly head-mistressy. In any event I couldn't delay James's appointment as it might prejudice his health.

I felt a sting of dismay. My feelings were less numb these days, they were slowly returning as if they had been frozen and were now thawing.

The sting really stung. There was my little son, whose skeleton was being gradually deformed by the pull of his own spastic muscles, and I couldn't even go to an appointment with his orthopaedic consultant. It was unthinkable. I felt tears well up and spill down my face.

With these feelings came an uncomfortable awareness that things didn't feel right. It wasn't surreal, as it had been when I was suicidally depressed. Then, I had felt as if I were playing a part on a stage set, which I could exit if I chose, by drowning myself. This time I felt real, but it was painful.

A tsunami had struck my life in 1999 when James had been born so early and brain damaged. A typhoon had followed it, one that lasted for years. Now I had realised that it was over, I could stop trying to cling to a tree. Instead I had to let go and survey the devastation it had caused.

I spoke to my wise friend Anna, who was a counsellor. I knew she wouldn't be able to take me as a client; I had to have someone who didn't know me. But, having looked at the multitude of people on the internet I could pay to listen to my problems, I was daunted. It was such a personal service. 'Do you know anyone I can go to?' I asked her. 'Someone who you think will get on with me?' 'There is one person I am thinking of', said Anna. 'She has a lot of experience.'

A week later I was being shown into a room with a big dark leather chair (for me). The counsellor was very blonde, radiant with health and her manner exuded calm. She sat on a smaller chair opposite me, with a silver tubular structure. I felt later that the chairs were symbolic of our different states of mind and body. I was still 4 st overweight from the tribunal hearing and full of dark unresolved emotions. She was slim, poised and projected a sense of inner peace. 'Why have you come to see me, Jane?' she asked.

I began to sob. 'Ten years ago I gave birth at 25 weeks to a little boy who is severely disabled,' I said. 'I feel as if I have been through a tsunami, and I am left with a beach full of wreckage. I don't know who I am any more.'

*

Out of the blue I received payments from the Council to cover a whole year's worth of carers for when James was home. I was overwhelmed. Surely they had got it wrong, it was too much! Social worker # 6 came to the house again and confirmed that the money was indeed correct.

I asked him what was happening with James's 48-week package at school and the First and Second Panels. He said that the manager was the one who had the best knowledge of the ins and outs of James's case, and I should get in touch with him soon as he was leaving. I was instantly alarmed. I remembered the advice of the independent reviewing officer that James's respite could be revoked at any time by a social care manager. It was the manager who had authorised James's respite. Now he was leaving. I wrote to him asking him to respond before he left and also asking for a meeting.

I never got a reply.

*

In October I went to see James for what were settling down to be twice-termly visits. I had developed a new emotional radar. I found that I could go for five weeks without missing him too much, but after that the umbilical cord tugged and I ached to hold him, to see his face, and just to be with him.

After some trial and error, I found a routine that suited us both. It was intensely draining being with James at Dame Hannah's, because I was seeing my child living in a different environment to home, getting close to other people who, while reassuringly loving, were doing things in a different way to me. I realised that if our being together there affected me so profoundly, what was it doing to James? I understood when I was going to come and go, but he didn't. I had yet to find a way of explaining the concept of time to him beyond five-minute countdowns: 5-4-3-2-1. The answer was to have a set routine so that he knew what to expect.

I found that it was best if I arrived at 2pm, when James was about to go back to school after lunch. The lunch break lasted from 12-2pm at Dame Hannah's to allow time for the students to eat and then rest. Many of them had complex medical needs that took time to deal with, such as suctioning their airways. All needed toileting. James didn't have medical needs but would sleep after he had eaten, as much to 'zone out' as anything. If I were there after lunch, he was too excited and couldn't relax.

I would take him over to school for the afternoon session, which gave me the opportunity to talk to his teachers and therapists and to hang out with him in a place that wasn't home, but where he was comfortable. There was no restriction on what I could do with James, as might have been the case with a mainstream school. I could stay with him all the time and take part in his therapy if I wanted. I could go on the trampoline with him and make him ask me for big bounces. I could go in the hydrotherapy pool or take him out of lessons to go swimming at the leisure centre. I would then go back to the bungalow where he lived in the grounds, and stay with him while he ate supper. After he had eaten, I would go. If I stayed on into the evening, he would become exhausted with emotion and so would I. If I left at 5.30pm, he could have a normal evening and calm down before bedtime. I could go back to my B&B and have a rare night without children, watching what I wanted on TV and reading the newspaper.

The next day I would come to the bungalow for 8.30am, have a cuddle then take James over to school for 9am. I would stay with him for morning school, then leave when he had eaten lunch and needed his sleep. In this way, he got used to the length of my visits, when they would start and when they would end. Gradually, over the next two years, the tension would seep out of them as they became routine.

I had to be careful though not to be seen by James if I wasn't going to be able to spend time with him. If I had said 'goodbye' but was seeing the teacher afterwards, I would have to hide around corners like a character from *The Pink Panther*, while James went by. If he saw me, he would want me to stay with him and if I didn't stay he would become upset and confused.

At the end of one particular visit, in October, I was driving out of the school just before 1pm. I put BBC Radio 4 on, and caught the familiar and rather cherished beeps. Beep, beep, beep, beep, beeeeeeeeeeeeeeeeeep. The very first headline said that an internal inquiry had found that Birmingham children's social care department was not fit for purpose.

I had only just pulled onto a dual carriageway and was merging with traffic going at over 70mph. I thought of myself as a careful driver. I nevertheless involuntarily punched the air and shouted at the top of my voice 'YESSSS!' Then I pulled into a lay-by and had a brief cry. I had had no idea that such an inquiry was going on. The fog of depression combined with the busy nature of my life had not left me capable of digging for information on a macro level about the Council's performance.

I suddenly realised the insidious effect that dealing with the Council over the years had had on me. I had become so used to dealing with a huge, ineffectual machine that I had come to anticipate that nothing would happen. I had become fatalistic about the services that James and I could expect. Now the machine had shown self-awareness! I was elated.

The feeling went far deeper than just a sense of justice that the failure of the system was being exposed. It was a relief that the democracy I had grown up in and valued, was still working. It wasn't as if the individual people I had dealt with at the Council had seemed anything other than compassionate and concerned. However, I had still developed the feeling that the organisation itself was at best chaotic and ineffectual and at worst, capricious.

The headline wasn't expanded upon in that news bulletin, but there were more details in the newspaper the next day. The inquiry had been carried out by the scrutiny committee of the Council.

The report, written by Councillor Len Clark, said:

'Preface

Many of the findings of this Inquiry report into children's social care may not make comfortable reading for the Council...

Unfortunately Birmingham's children's social care service has a history of underperformance over the past decade...

Fundamentally addressing these very serious concerns in respect of children's social care services in Birmingham must finally be an issue of priorities for the Cabinet. Failure to tackle these issues will mean that our most vulnerable children and families pay a heavy price...

Summary

... Our findings demonstrated an extremely fragile management structure and the inevitable conclusion is that the current social work model is not fit for purpose.' [23]

Later that month I received James's annual report from Dame Hannah's, listing his educational achievements and once again I was left with a full heart. I couldn't believe the care and expertise that went into the curriculum for the children.

The physiotherapist had recommended a special chair for James to use in the classroom. It would mean he could be out of his wheelchair during lessons.

His teachers had described his activities.

'The theme for the Spring term 2009 was 'Elements'. James... has been learning how to make toast and butter. The bread is frozen so this enables him to learn that the toaster changes it from very cold to hot. He helps to spread the butter and experiences it melting. Just before Easter he melted chocolate whilst helping to make Easter eggs and nests. James was very keen on the chocolate, both solid and melted! He explored the properties of ice in several ways, for instance, we told the story of Titanic in a multi-sensory way using a computer slideshow,

[23] *'Who Cares? Protecting Children and Improving Children's Social care',* a report by the Overview and Scrutiny Committee of Birmingham City Council, 13 October 2009.

music and various props. James liked touching the 'iceberg' floating in a bowl of water best...'

I noted all of the things that James could now do, after 18 months at Dame Hannah's, which he hadn't done before.

He was now learning to use the toilet; he could get in and out of his wheelchair with just a little help, and was learning to drive a powered chair. He could make several signs with his hand, hold a pen and drink from an open cup. He could also get on and off his bed with just a little help, use a touch-screen computer, clean his teeth with his own toothbrush with help, use a trike, and tolerate listening to stories in a group situation.

It wasn't that his Birmingham school had failed him. On the contrary, it was an award-winning school. It was just that it wasn't open 24 hours a day and James hadn't had one-to-one staff allocated to him there.

We had a letter from his funny houseparent.

*'Now then I have a very little confession well actually it is big confession.................Like I said James was ill with a cold so yesterday morning we went into the sensory room. Well......
It's a lovely quiet room soft lights, nice and warm and James snuggled up and he had a pillow and I just may have snuggled with him..........can you see where this is going? ......well James fell asleep ....and well........I may have closed my eyes for a second.........well it just may have been a little more than a second......let's just say James and I had a very nice morning nap.....How embarrassing!!! It was the talk of the class...'*

*

In November it was time for James's CIC review and also his annual education review. They were held together for the benefit of the staff travelling from Birmingham. Social worker # 6 was there, together with the independent reviewing officer. I found it hard not to adopt a mock parrot voice as I repeated yet again the catalogue of attempts to clarify James's package at Dame Hannah's. The school staff who attended were horrified.

In the minutes of the meeting the independent reviewing officer stated that both he and the social worker would take up the matter of James's placement. He wrote:

'3. [Independent reviewing officer] to email the Team Manager and Operations Manager at the Children's Disabilities Team regarding funding of James's placement.

4. Social Worker to convey Mrs Raca's concerns regarding the funding issues surrounding James's placement with his Team Manager'.

Both actions were marked to be done as soon as possible. Nothing happened.

That year, Dame Hannah's had decided to stay open for 52 weeks, so for the first time we had the option to leave James there for Christmas itself. It didn't take long for me to make a decision. It was almost impossible for us to get a carer to come home with James at Christmas. He wasn't interested in presents and wouldn't eat with us. All it meant for him was a house full of excited busy people, who had even less time than usual to spend with him. If he stayed at Dame Hannah's he would have a James-based Christmas. Santa Claus would come and bring suitable presents and he would have someone to look after just him for the whole day.

It sounded lovely. If I had no other family than him I should have loved a Dame Hannah's Christmas myself. But I had two other children and extended family obligations to fulfil. I booked James's homecoming for the week he broke up, with a return the day before Christmas Eve.

After two days at home he had a seizure which was so bad we had to call the paramedics. By the time he left to go back to Dame Hannah's, I was wrung out with emotion and sleeplessness.

I hadn't had time to prepare anything, so Christmas Eve passed in a blur of present wrapping, making up beds for guests and wishing, for yet another year, that I had had time to cook.

*

In 2009, central government issued an improvement notice to Birmingham City Council due to:

'...poor performance/decline in: Children's social care and safeguarding...' [24]

An unannounced Ofsted inspection found that:

'The range of services for children in need and their families who require more intensive multi-agency support but are not in need of child protection is too limited. This contributes to high referral rates to children's social care and unmet need as some serious cases are not diverted to relevant family support provision'. [25]

Ofsted's annual rating for children's services in Birmingham City Council 2009 found that it performed poorly. [26]

[24] Improvement Notice, Department of Children Schools and Families to Birmingham City Council, 10 February 2009.

[25] Annual unannounced inspection of contact, referral and assessment arrangements within Birmingham City Council children's services, Ofsted 9 December 2009.

[26] Children's services annual rating, Birmingham City Council, Ofsted, 9 December 2009.

Chapter 13
PEACE
2010

As our new way of life slowly began to settle down, I noticed how much I loved visiting James at his school, in contrast to dreading his visits home. I was able to do things with him that I could never do in Birmingham, because he would tolerate going out on trips in Devon. I could go with him on a group outing with the other children, or anywhere I chose, with the help of a carer. I took him to the beach, even in the winter, putting him in an old wetsuit. He knelt at the edge of the sea, as he had done after his first term at Dame Hannah's. His face was once again pure ecstasy as he lifted it to the wind and the weak winter sun. He swept his fingers across the icy wet sand and gasped at the feel of the cold white surf.

When we got back to the bungalow, in the specially adapted school van, we put him straight into a big hot deep bath full of bubbles. It was like an armchair with a door in front. James sat on a seat in the middle while the water rose up to his waist. He had sand everywhere, even in his ears.

Our afternoon routine, whether it was a weekend or a school day, included a cuddle on his bed in the bungalow. He had a TV on the wall (put out of his reach by the handymen), and we would snuggle up to watch *Postman Pat*. Mercifully, *Teletubbies* was now so out of date that there were no DVDs of them in the bungalow.

James still had a nasty habit of trying to get into his pad and had long since found out how to get into the bathing type suits I had commissioned for him from a local dancewear company. I made do for a while with some large sunsuits from the supermarket – the sort that protect toddlers on the beach, with long sleeves, legs below the knee and a zip up the front. James had to have a girl's one in pastel pink, since it was the only one left in his size. I hoped that his gender identity wasn't sufficiently formed for him to mind.

After a while the sunsuits fell apart, so I did some research and found there was now something I could buy called a 'Houdini' suit, a name which made me smile.

This was like a giant babygro with a zip up the back. For a while it solved the problem, until James worked out that he could gnaw holes in it and get his hand in that way. The most dangerous time for him to be wearing a holey Houdini suit was at night when he was on his own, waking at odd times. However, his nights had begun to improve after the occupational therapist had him assessed by a sleep counsellor, who put in place some new routines.

I had heard nothing from anyone about James's 48-week jointly funded placement. I was anxious to resolve it.

Apart from wanting his holiday provision to be secure and not revoked at the whim of one manager, I wanted it to be increased from 46 weeks and 4 days to 48 weeks. James had to come home for seven days at a time, but I was finding that his visits became almost intolerable for all of us after five days. This was because he still only tolerated a very limited existence at home, compared to school. He would only go out to a few familiar places and still insisted on remaining in the playroom when at home and watching *Teletubbies*. After five days he became bored and aggressive and the carer and I were exhausted. If I could increase his placement to 48 weeks he would only ever need to come home for five days at a time.

On one occasion when James had been home for seven days, a neighbour rang the doorbell. The carer was on a break and I was responsible for James on my own.

I rushed to answer the door, then immediately told the neighbour to follow me back into the hall, where James was going for a stroll in his walker.

As she entered the house, she saw James tipping over a vase of flowers so the water went all over the carpet, and then he grabbed and ate a tulip. We managed to get the tulip out of his mouth by doing a countdown '5-4-3-2-1'. He would become still when he heard this, and on the count of 1 he usually cooperated. On this occasion, however, after handing us the tulip he then turned and started trying to pull a picture off the wall. It was a wine map of France which I had had framed for Andrew's birthday many years earlier, and which was precious to both of us. I managed to wrest it off him without breaking the glass or getting bitten. James immediately turned his attention to a photograph of Elizabeth. The neighbour, who hadn't seen James for some years, was so taken aback by what she saw that I had to prompt her as to why she had come.

Sometimes James's boredom would tip over into aggression. He usually reserved this for people he knew well, but not always. On another occasion he took a swipe at a visiting social worker. He was now tall enough to reach light switches by kneeling up and strong enough to break your arm if he chose.

I was sorry for the social worker but thought it was rather useful for her to see his behaviour at first hand.

I spoke to my councillor again, who suggested taking the matter of James's placement up with the director of children's services. I decided to follow her advice. I hadn't realised that there was one director who was in charge of both the education and social care departments of the Council, when it came to children. My experience of the two departments was that they were in two different buildings several miles apart. In my mind the physical separation was mirrored by the administrative separation which I had experienced.

I wrote a letter to the director, recording my attempts to get a 48-week placement agreed by the First Panel and the Second Panel. Since the tribunal, I had made a point of putting all my communications with the Council in writing, in case I later needed them as evidence. I waited for an answer to my letter. It was to be another 15 months before I got one.

I also wrote to the education department of the Council. At James's annual review four months earlier, the physiotherapist had recommended that he should have a special classroom chair. I wanted to know what had happened about it. I got a reply saying they had passed the request on to health:

'We are currently liaising with Health regarding the request for funding of a chair for James. You will be informed of the outcome when they have informed us of how they wish to proceed.'

I contacted the education department twice more, to be told they were still waiting to hear from health.

At James's next annual review that autumn (almost one year after the chair had been recommended), the head teacher said that education had called him during the summer holidays to say that they would now fund the chair if they could agree a financial contribution by Dame Hannah's. However, by that time, the physiotherapist had assessed James's knees as now too stiff for the chair to be appropriate. During those months of wrangling over who would pay for the chair, James's legs had grown and changed.

We were lucky in that James was pretty healthy and robust, considering his disabilities. He didn't need oxygen, wasn't tube fed and wasn't immobile. Many of the children at the school were, and they were very vulnerable, hence the availability of nursing care 24 hours a day. One very sad consequence was that from time to time one of the children died. In this year, by pure coincidence, two students died on the same night.

Dame Hannah's is such a close community that everyone there was devastated. I thought of the fights those bereaved families may have had, to get equipment and support for their children. I often spoke to other parents and knew from anecdotal evidence that there was a universal battle to get help from local authorities and health services. It seemed so unquestionable to me that there should be no delay in obtaining it. There should be a clear, open pathway for children like James. What higher priority for state spending could there be?

*

In February it was Tom's birthday. Tom was into geography, so Elizabeth and I had spent hours making a cake in the shape of the British Isles, with Smarties demarcating the major cities. As a precaution, we put the cake at the opposite end of the table to where James was sitting and went to get Tom, the birthday boy. As we returned, we saw that James had pulled the tablecloth and was cunningly reeling in the cake towards him. He was about to plunge his greedy hand into Cardiff when Lucy, who had returned from her travels, grabbed it just in time.

For Elizabeth's birthday the following month, I was commissioned to make a seaside cake. After creating a harbour with blocks of Battenberg, we used two bottles of blue colouring to make a marzipan sea, and then stuck freshly washed bath toys such as boats and sharks into it. One toy was a miniature doll with a missing arm. We both decided that a disabled swimmer was entirely appropriate, and so into the blue marzipan she went, positioned into a one-armed front crawl.

At Easter, when James came home, he took part in the Passion play at church. Each year, the children from Sunday school put on a rather chaotic but enjoyable production, designed to teach them about the Crucifixion. James and Edmund, the vicar's autistic son, were always included. On this occasion James played Pontius Pilate with a splendid laurel wreath. The laurel leaves were real and as James has a taste for greenery, there wasn't much of it left by the time Jesus was being sentenced.

The following term, James got his own electric wheelchair. It was supplied by a charity as the Council only provided his manual one. The staff were very excited because if he could learn to use it well, it would give him independence.

I had grieved for James's inability to walk for many years. Watching my little boy full of energy but not able to run about, caused me unbearable anguish. From time to time this surfaced in my dreams, but there was joy mixed with the pain. I would dream that he was racing around and talking to me as if he weren't disabled in any way. He was always on a green hillside in the sunshine (the influence of *Teletubbies* no doubt), wearing a light blue T-shirt. The joy came because my mind was able to produce a completely real image of him without any of his disabilities. It wasn't only physically real – it was James with all his character. Nothing he said was a surprise because I already knew him. He was witty and cheeky, outrageous and selfish, loving and affectionate. The dreams were a little glimpse of heaven. Waking to see them for what they were was painful. I grieved for Tom then, having seen more fully the brother he would never climb trees with, ride bikes with or have a pint with.

The electric chair would enable James to decide where he wanted to go and to do it himself. It was a significant leap forward from being pushed by a carer. In his electric chair he might decide, for example, that he wanted to visit the school kitchen, and off he could go. I didn't envy the kitchen staff an impromptu visit from James. They would have to hide all the food.

James's houseparent got very excited about the electric chair.

'Today has been stunning James had ago in the powered wheelchair. He has only been in this a few times but WOW he is soooooooooooo learning how to work that joystick. Today he drove into Debs office with purpose he really wanted to go and see her. He managed to get himself through the door!!!!! And steer himself around a sofa. Debs and I were so proud of him. He managed to turn around leave her room and then drove up to the kitchen where I gave him some grapes. What a star and soooooooooooo clever as it is very difficult to drive an electric wheel chair.'

One of his favourite places to go was the laundry. The ladies there spoiled him and he loved to watch the washing machines go round and round.

When I next visited him, I saw him having a session in the new chair. We started off in the school hall. There were two exits, one leading directly outside, and the other leading down the main corridor. The carer intended James to go straight outside. James had other ideas. Firstly, he drove towards an internal wall. I thought he was trying to crash on purpose, but he was aiming at a board with symbols stuck on with Velcro. He picked a symbol off the board, drove over to the carer and gave it to her, then turned around and went out of the hall down the main corridor. The symbol was a picture of an empty square and said 'gone'. He was off on an expedition of his own choosing.

We followed James down the main corridor, past reception and out of the front entrance to the school. He went along a path that came to a fork, with a bush in the middle. 'Which way do you want to go James?' I asked, 'Left or right?' James's answer was to drive straight into the bush. I thought he had lost control of the chair and leapt forward, but he had simply decided he wanted to taste the bush. I realised with humility that James knew perfectly well what he wanted and was no fool when it came to his own safety. He just didn't see the world the same way that other people did, nor did he feel the need to conform. I felt an enormous respect for him, similar to the emotion I had felt when he first stood up in the shower at home eight years earlier.

*

The 2010 general election was called. My councillor knocked on the door and we had a brief chat. I told her I had not had a reply to my letter to the director of children's services about James's placement, sent many weeks earlier. 'Isn't it awful?!' she said.

In anticipation of the election, a letter signed by 30 charities and patient groups was published, attacking the Labour Government's record on health.

It said that money which had been given to local authorities to fund, among other things, respite breaks for disabled children, had not been ring-fenced. As a result, much of it had been used for other purposes. [27] I thought of an interview I had given to BBC Radio West Midlands in 2007, when the Government announced it was making £340 million available for respite breaks for disabled children. I had said then that although it sounded like a great deal of money, it probably wasn't enough as there was so much need out there. Now it seemed that even that funding had not all reached its intended destination.

In May there was the usual CIC review. This one was attended by another new social worker, # 7, as social worker # 6 was on sick leave.

We got chatting and I asked her whether there was a separate team dealing with children in need of protection, or whether those social workers dealt with children in need as well. She said that the majority of her case load was

27 *Laura Donnelly, The Telegraph online, 17 April 2010.*

dealing with children in need of protection. She had spent most of the previous day in court on a child protection case. The social care manager at the tribunal over two years earlier had said that the two sorts of work would be handled in future by different teams, but plainly that wasn't happening.

At the CIC review, I repeated what I had said at the previous review, about James's 46-week and 4-day placement needing to be jointly funded by education, health and social care, and for it to be 48 weeks.

The independent reviewing officer told the social worker that she would need to discuss this with her team manager and inform me of the result. This was to be actioned 'As soon as possible'.

I appreciated the independent reviewing officer's sense of urgency. However, I didn't believe anything would happen as a result of what she had said. The same recommendation in one form or another had been made at every LAC and CIC review for almost 2 years and nothing had changed.

I decided that it was ridiculous to have these six-monthly meetings to discuss James's health and wellbeing if a critical issue such as the length and security of his placement at a children's home remained unresolved. I asked the independent reviewing officer if she had any authority to censure the Council or to bring pressure to bear on them. She said that she didn't.

What, I thought, was the use of the Council employing these independent reviewing officers if they had no teeth?

Then the independent reviewing officer said that what I needed was an advocate. She said the Council provided an advocacy service for children like James.

Privately I thought I was capable of doing my own advocacy in this matter. But then I thought that the advocate might have an inside knowledge of the Council's labyrinthine systems; he just might make something happen. I accepted the offer. The next I heard, the advocate, someone I had never met, had been to visit James at Dame

219

Hannah's without telling me. I discovered that he was there to be 'James's voice'. His remit was to find out what James wanted in all this! I was alarmed and cross. I didn't need someone else telling me what James thought and felt.

I did realise though, that we had a good package for James and that, provided it continued, we had almost all we had asked for.

One evening I paused on the landing to gaze at the sunset. The sky looked completely still. It was golden where the orb of the sun was sitting on the rooftops but this faded to pink and then violet, as I looked upwards. The whole picture was streaked with unmoving clouds.

The tranquillity and beauty of what I was seeing reflected a peace which I had begun to feel inside me. I realised that despite the continuing issues over James's placement and the emotional pain of his separation, I had come to terms with it.

I had begun to hear the bird song in the garden. It was as if the birds had stopped singing for a few years and then begun again. I would take a minute to pause and enjoy the smell of newly cut grass when Andrew mowed the lawn. I had been so trapped inside both my own head and my own house that for years I had stopped hearing and seeing those things. I also noticed that now I laughed more freely and more often.

I was still seeing the serene counsellor, but only once a month instead of weekly. At first I had cried every time we met, but after a few weeks there were visits when I left without having wept. These occasions became more and more frequent.

I realised that I had been working very hard for years, just to keep all of us going. Life had been polarised between the domestic drudgery involved in running a large family and the high drama of James's condition. The bit in between had been left out. I hadn't had time to absorb what had happened to me – to all of us. There had been an emotional backlog of 11 years to work through.

The backlog had also applied to our paperwork. The piles on the floor gradually went down. In the process I found tax returns that hadn't been filed, insurance claim forms that had never been filled in, and letters from the bank that had never been answered. I had several years' worth of Christmas cards with details of people's change of address and the names of their newly born children, which I had intended to make a note of one day.

As the piles of paper went down, so did my weight. I felt rather like Nanny McPhee, who started off looking like a giantess and shrank as she imposed order around her.

*

We continued to get letters from Dame Hannah's, allowing us into James's new and full life:

'*Hiya all.*

…James joined his friends on Monday evening chilling out and watching post-man pat. James also made some chocolate buns CHIEF TASTER. James also enjoyed a hand and foot massage and made his choice signing really liked his foot massage'.

'*We went to B and Q for life skills, I bet you are thinking Lovely!!!!!!!!! Maybe with a hint of sarcasm? Well James loved it. I think the reason being, it was a HUGE shop, very light and airy, with really big aisles and soft music playing in the background the aim was to look at different building materials. So James had a feel of stone, cement and soft and hard materials. We also read lots of signs as James is working hard on a lot of his letters.*'

'*Yesterday we went to the library, it was soooooooooo good. . James held out his hand and signed hello to the librarian, which was amazing. I think we managed a photo of this. It was moving to watch….*'

Just before Dame Hannah's broke up in July, they held their first ever prom for the students. I sent a black tie outfit for James, consisting of a pair of old school trousers, a black jacket from a charity shop and one of Andrew's black ties from our London years. The school sent back a picture of James next to a cream-coloured Rolls Royce, looking like a disabled James Bond with his dickie bow.

He wouldn't have gone to an evening prom in Birmingham.

*

In the summer I went to visit James while the World Cup was on. It was an afternoon when England was playing and the whole country had gone indoors to watch. I took James swimming in the leisure centre near Dame Hannah's and we had the pool to ourselves. The only other person in there was the life guard perched on top of his high stepladder. He was straining to see the match on the TV in the café, which he could just glimpse through the window. He looked disgruntled about having to be on duty at such a pivotal time.

It was a very hot day and we spent a long time in the pool, with James deciding to lick the entire perimeter. It was the best swim we had ever had, as with no one else there I didn't have to worry about James trying to assault them. We floated companionably around, meeting up every now and then for a 'chloriney' kiss. I watched the sunlight dance on the blue water and enjoyed just feeling happy.

So many years had passed when I had not felt happy at just being alive. I had come to savour happy moments now – to recognise them and hold them for a while before time moved them on.

Later in the summer, James came home to Birmingham for his usual visit. On this occasion he startled me by learning how to use his 'up and down' bed, which the occupational therapist had finally obtained. It had a motor underneath so that I could raise James up high to change his pad, but could lower it to the ground at night so he could get on and off with ease.

I came in one morning to find him perched 4 ft in the air, looking down at me as if on some magic carpet and giggling. My heart was in my mouth – he could have fallen off! After that the power was turned off at night.

We had begun to celebrate his birthdays properly. He had become used to parties at Dame Hannah's and was far less overwhelmed by them than he had been in the past. We all went to see *Toy Story 3* at the cinema, one of the few places he would tolerate going. When we got home we were just about to tuck into his party food when he had a seizure. Now that my feelings were working again, I didn't just feel cold, dull and resigned. I felt the adrenaline of panic and the sadness of a lost celebration. My poor little suffering boy.

We were visited by yet another social worker, # 8. She was very friendly and competent. She still took out a blank pad though and asked me to tell her about James. I asked whether there was anything on their system she could read instead of me repeating ten years' worth of history. She told me that there was some information, but unfortunately her predecessors hadn't all loaded their notes onto the system as they should have done. She invited me to email her any documents I wanted, so she could put them onto what was called the 'care first' system. In the meantime she had requested James's paper files from storage. I did contemplate emailing her all my correspondence but then calculated it would take me about a month to do it. So I gave up.

In November, there was a bonfire party at the vicarage. It was on a Thursday night when Edmund was at his weekly boarding school so he wasn't home. There were fireworks, wine, food and music. After a while I realised that the atmosphere in the house was very different to when Edmund was around. There was a sense of elation and release in Joanna and the vicar. I told Joanna this and she pulled a face. She told me that when he was home, Edmund had started to use their bed as a toilet! I suggested this was quite a compliment, a gesture of love, and she agreed, but she was fed up with washing the sheets.

James came home for part of the Christmas holidays again. It was particularly difficult to occupy him in winter, when we couldn't go outside easily. We could, however, take him to church. Apart from the Passion play at Easter, where he had starred as Pontius Pilate, there was also the children's Christmas play. This was put on every year, and since a little bit of chaos was the order of the day, it made me feel more comfortable when James started grabbing the flower displays. Edmund took part and his behaviour was a trifle unconventional too.

This Christmas, James was in the starring role of Joseph. I pushed him along the aisle in his wheelchair, hoping he wouldn't try to grab Mary as we processed towards the stable. Instead he ate his words, literally, chewing the piece of paper with his lines on until it was a soggy lump. Now I didn't have the sheet telling me who was saying what and when! Fortunately I had a reasonable idea of the story, so we could improvise. The attention wasn't on me and James anyway, as Edmund ran amok, blowing out the Advent candles. Elizabeth stayed serenely in the pulpit, being an exemplary narrator. Tom wasn't there as he had decided he was an atheist.

After Christmas we had the deepest snow in the UK for decades. The Council cancelled the minibus which had been booked to take James and Lucy, the carer, back to Devon. The transport department assessed it to be too dangerous to make the journey. Although I was dismayed at first, a long look at the weather forecast for Devon persuaded me they were right. Lucy had to go back by hook or crook though, so we faced being snowed in with James for days, with no help.

The prospect was appalling and I was determined to get James back any way possible, if it were safe to do so. The trains were in chaos but the main lines still seemed to be running, so James had his first train journey, travelling from Birmingham to Plymouth. He was given a wheelchair space in first class, endless free biscuits and thoroughly enjoyed himself. Elizabeth and I ended up escorting him and Lucy as far as Cheltenham, since in the mêlée at the station the train left with no announcement and us still on it. We hammered on the window while the train was still in the station, but the doors had locked and the guards could do nothing. Elizabeth burst into tears at the shock of it, but I just laughed. Compared to past traumas it was nothing. We passed the time playing charades, and soon she was laughing too.

I had still not had a substantive response to the letter I had sent by recorded delivery to the director of children's services in January. It was now December. I had been asking him to confirm that James's whole placement at Dame Hannah's was funded by health, education and social care, so that it couldn't just be revoked by one social care manager. I had also been asking him to increase it from 46 weeks and 4 days to 48 weeks. Between us the councillor and I had sent six letters/emails chasing for a response and had received no fewer than six holding responses from a variety of different people. One person had written in his email:

'...*my secretary is on leave but i will try and identify what letter you are awaiting a response to......... but it does seem you have been waiting a long time. can you remind me please?*'

This was going nowhere. I had to do something about it, but there was no social care tribunal to go to. I found out I could go to the local government ombudsman and the councillor gave me a leaflet. I read that before I went to

225

the ombudsman I should go through the Council's official complaints procedure. I realised that the Council had a whole customer relations department, just like Sainsbury's!

I filed a complaint and an independent investigating officer (not to be confused with an independent reviewing officer) sat in my kitchen with a laptop and made a detailed note. I told him the facts I had been repeating to the Council and to anyone who would listen for over two years. He grew grave. His report was sent to me four months later, by a new manager at the disabled children's team.

My complaint had been split into eight parts and the investigator had upheld all of them. The new manager who sent me the report wrote a long and articulate letter apologising on behalf of the Council:

'It is absolutely imperative that I acknowledge that your complaints extend over an exceptionally long period. I apologise on behalf of the team and the service and for the decision making processes which have conspicuously failed to address your issues and give you a clear decision or communicate effectively with you.

...It is clear to me that the communications with you about James' and the family's needs were not handled in an appropriate manner. Also the actions following on from the various panel meetings were not followed. Throughout all of these processes from a number of different sections of the service you have received poor or no communication. Overall it is easy to see that the Directorate have not communicated with in [sic] an appropriate manner.'

He had also ensured that the Second Panel considered James's 46 weeks and 4 days placement. As far as I understood it, the members had agreed that this should be tripartite funded so now it was officially an overall package.

At last, after nearly three years, he had his package. But they weren't going to give us 48 weeks.

I decided to give in.

The receipt of an apology and an indication that someone was finally taking control of the situation at the Council had pricked the balloon of my anger and it was gradually beginning to deflate. Perhaps it was also something to do with my sessions with the serene counsellor, but a few months after I received that letter I felt myself letting the balloon go altogether and watching it drift slowly away.

*

One morning I sat in the kitchen and read the latest letter from James's houseparent.

'Yesterday I worked from 11am–10pm I took your little man sailing oh my gosh I was expecting a sail in a boat and just a little jaunt on the water. Soooooo wrong. We actually went sailing the real mcCoy we went to Teignmouth. From start to finish the day was just astounding. The men involved were just lush, kind, men, explaining to James, every step of the way what they were doing... they lifted James in his wheelchair and escorted me onto one boat where we had to go to a pontoon ...then they lifted James into the sailing boat. James was calm, happy, even signing yes and please.

We...are in the sailing boat it had a huge sail that we had to duck under several times when it leaned on its side. James was beaming and trailing his hand in the sea... I forgot to say James was lifted out of his wheelchair and is strapped into his own seat. We were sailing for about an hour. Just stunning. We had sun, wind, it was a bit emotional really...'

My little boy had been sailing!

The school was going to try to raise funds to buy its own adapted boat, so eventually he might be able to go out on the sea all the time.

I looked out of the window at the climbing frame that James had never been able to climb.

It didn't hurt so much any more.

*

In July 2010 a joint inspection by Ofsted and the Care Quality Commission found that children's services at Birmingham City Council were inadequate overall in the area of safeguarding children in need of protection. [28] Central government issued a second improvement notice in relation to this. [29]

In December 2010 Ofsted produced its Annual Children's Services Assessment. It graded children's services at Birmingham as performing poorly. [30]

[28] *Inspection of safeguarding and looked after children services: Birmingham. Ofsted/Care Quality Commission, 16 July 2010.*
[29] *Improvement Notice, Department of Education to Birmingham City Council, 30 September 2010.*
[30] *Annual children's services assessment, Birmingham City Council children's services, Ofsted, 9 December 2010.*

AFTERWORD

In November 2011 Ofsted produced its Annual Children's Services Assessment. It graded children's services at Birmingham as performing poorly. [31] The report stated that :

'Birmingham has in place an improvement plan to address ... identified weaknesses and is making progress in line with this...However the children's services assessment for 2011 remains poorly until further safeguarding inspection evidence is available.

The weaknesses in safeguarding services are significant...'

ACKNOWLEDGEMENTS

My sincere thanks to Rosa Monckton, who campaigns tirelessly for disabled children, for agreeing to write a foreword. My warmest thanks also to Susannah Straughan, my editor and friend, and to the following people, who were instrumental in helping me to take this book out of my head and put it onto paper.

Karen Butler	Anne Lavery
Helen Fenton	Debbie Sargant
Averil Heaton	Katherine Tamlyn
John and Lesley Heaton	Carolyn Tatman
Yvonne Jones	Sandy Ward

My warmest thanks also to the following people for being guinea pigs and/or for their help and advice.

Dr Anne Aukett	Sarah Molloy
Dr Jeff Bissenden	Lucy Rayner
Lisa Clark	Jane Ridge
Ilona Curtis	Dr Helen Robertson
Miss Gabrielle Downey	Deborah Robinson
Mrs Andrea Jester	Dr Andy Tatman
Anne Lamb	Fiona Taylor
Lauren Marchant	Joanna Tomlinson

And most of all to Andrew, Tom and Elizabeth for putting up with me disappearing for hours to write, and then appearing and talking endlessly about disability.

ABOUT THE AUTHOR

Jane Raca lives in Birmingham with her husband, Andrew, and two, sometimes three, of their children.
After writing this book for three years, she is taking a break before deciding what to do next. She is passionate about improving provision for disabled children.

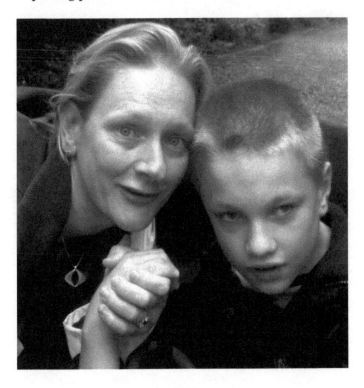

www.standingupforjames.co.uk